FLIPPING THE NURSING CLASSROOM

Where Active Learning Meets Technology

Karen Hessler, PhD, RN, FNP-C
Associate Professor
College of Health and Human Science
School of Nursing
University of Northern Colorado

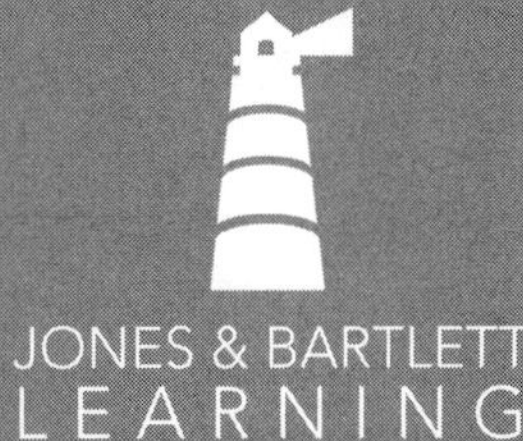

World Headquarters
Jones & Bartlett Learning
5 Wall Street
Burlington, MA 01803
978-443-5000
info@jblearning.com
www.jblearning.com

Jones & Bartlett Learning books and products are available through most bookstores and online booksellers. To contact Jones & Bartlett Learning directly, call 800-832-0034, fax 978-443-8000, or visit our website, www.jblearning.com.

Substantial discounts on bulk quantities of Jones & Bartlett Learning publications are available to corporations, professional associations, and other qualified organizations. For details and specific discount information, contact the special sales department at Jones & Bartlett Learning via the above contact information or send an email to specialsales@jblearning.com.

Production Credits
VP, Executive Publisher: David D. Cella
Executive Editor: Amanda Martin
Associate Acquisitions Editor: Rebecca Myrick
Editorial Assistant: Danielle Bessette
Production Manager: Carolyn Rogers Pershouse
Production Editor: Vanessa Richards
Production Assistant: Rebecca Humphrey
Senior Marketing Manager: Jennifer Scherzay
Product Fulfillment Manager: Wendy Kilborn
Composition: S4Carlisle Publishing Services
Cover Design: Kristin E. Parker
Rights & Media Specialist: Merideth Tumasz
Media Development Editor: Troy Liston
Cover Image: © ra2studio/Shutterstock
Printing and Binding: Edwards Brothers Malloy
Cover Printing: Edwards Brothers Malloy

To order this product, use ISBN: 9781284101577

Library of Congress Cataloging-in-Publication Data
Names: Hessler, Karen, author.
Title: Flipping the nursing classroom : where active learning meets technology / Karen Hessler.
Description: Burlington, MA : Jones & Bartlett Learning, [2017] | Includes bibliographical references.
Identifiers: LCCN 2016001281 | ISBN 9781284109986
Subjects: | MESH: Education, Nursing—methods | Faculty, Nursing—standards | Models, Educational
Classification: LCC RT90 | NLM WY 18 | DDC 610.73071/1—dc23 LC record available at http://lccn.loc.gov/2016001281

6048

Printed in the United States of America
20 19 18 17 16 10 9 8 7 6 5 4 3 2 1

DEDICATION

The time and effort put into this book required perhaps the biggest sacrifice—time away from my family. To my wonderful and loving husband, Japheth, and beautiful children, Jackson and Madison—thank you for giving mom time to write. Your support, understanding, and love mean everything to me.

To Katherine (Kat) Johnson—thank you for pioneering the flipped classroom with me. I have learned so much working with you and revere our friendship.

To God—who inspires all, gives each of us a creative mind to do our work, and fosters hope and joy within each willing heart.

CONTENTS

REWORD

by Jon Bergman

The flipped classroom model has surprised me. When Aaron Sams and I pioneered the model in our high school science classes in 2007 we had no idea that it would grow into a global movement. At first we thought it was a great idea for math and science teaching, but didn't see the model's application in other content areas. However, as we continued to share the model, we met amazing educators who took the flipped classroom and applied it to virtually every subject area and grade level. Educators in the fields of kindergarten, English, social studies, physical education, auto mechanics, art, band, and, yes, nursing, have embraced the flipped class model. In the course of the past few years, I have had the chance to meet many nursing educators who are flipping their classes. I have noticed that nursing educators have been some of the quickest to adopt the model. I think the practical nature of nurses has propelled them to be early adopters.

Many years ago, Aaron Sams and I were presenting about the flipped classroom to a group of teachers and afterward one teacher came up to chat. She told us she was sold on the flipped model and wanted to start. She then paused and asked, "But what will I do in class now?" You see, all she had ever done was lecture and she did not know what she could do during class time if she flipped. Out of that conversation we realized that the flipped class starts with one simple question: "What is the best use of face-to-face class time?" The beauty of this question is that there is no "right" answer. This answer varies by subject matter, level, and even teacher disposition.

To that end, Karen Hessler has wrestled with this question in her context as a nursing professor. She has also thought about it in the broader context of good teaching and pedagogy. Karen has written this remarkable book, which dissects how flipped learning applies to nursing education. She draws on both research and her experiences as she flipped her own classes, to provide an excellent resource for nursing educators. I particularly like the many examples and practical tips Karen includes, which will help nursing educators start flipping their own classes in a short amount of time. She emphasizes how flipping her classes helps students move beyond information, and get them to apply what they have learned into the real-world job of being a nurse. In this world where there is such an emphasis on technology, which often seems to distance people from each other, Karen shares how flipping her classes brought her closer to her students. She realizes that good teaching, and nursing, is always best done in the context of positive relationships with students.

For those of you hesitant to try flipping your classes, I encourage you to take the time to read this book and consider how flipped learning can make your nursing classes more active and engaging. Learn from Karen's research, practical advice, and real-world stories. This book will challenge you to rethink how you have always taught and for many, it is my hope that this book will completely transform your teaching practice. So dive in and embrace flipped learning.

PREFACE

Nurse educators have historically been early adopters of new and innovative pedagogies in order to strengthen their ability to teach nursing students in the most efficacious and applicable manner. The flipped classroom approach to teaching and learning is no different. Several nurse educators across the country in both undergraduate and graduate nursing programs have tried their hand at using the method. Some early adopters of the method have had enough forethought to add an element of data collection and measurement to their implementation of the method as well. Podium and workshop sessions at nurse educator conferences have informed colleagues of individual applications of the method, including their specific results and advice for fellow flipping educators. However, a text that fully described the pedagogy of the flipped classroom, the research available on its use, and the ideas about a formalized process for implementation of the flipped classroom specific to nursing education was missing. This text was created to address the lack of a formal text for nurse educators interested in flipping their classrooms. It was also developed to help those nurse educators who had tried flipping the classroom with marginal or even negative results.

The book was also a result of many discussions with colleagues at conferences where I had presented on the flipped classroom for nursing education. Nursing educators asked for more than the handouts that they were given at the conference or pre-session workshops. Colleagues made it clear that they desired and needed more information about the flipped classroom. They wanted a book. Experience with the method in conjunction with consumption of the most current research lead to some solid notions about the flipped classroom as it could be applied specifically to our world of nursing education. The book seeks to provide those nursing educators desiring to flip their classroom with ideas, a template, and some direction in order to maximize success.

The first chapter of the book makes a case for the flipped classroom as an appropriate teaching strategy for nursing education. The most applicable and current research about the flipped classroom use in nursing is available within Chapter 2. Chapter 3 offers a conceptual model for planning, implementation, and evaluation of the flipped classroom for nurse educators. Chapters 4 through 8 focus on the different sections of the model and dive deeper into the actual application of the method within a nursing classroom. The final chapter is comprised of exemplars of nurse educators who have successfully flipped their classrooms. I hope the book, the suggestions, and the ideas within will augment teaching and learning in nursing education, and be an inspiration for flipping nursing educators everywhere.

CHAPTER 1

Why Flip the Nursing Classroom?

Introduction

Nursing educators are so innovative and imaginative, true explorers on the landscape of the profession of nursing. I have learned so much from those before me, and as a result, I am eager to share some of my knowledge in return. When I think of the professors that took me under their wing, I am so thankful that I have had so many excellent nurses showing me how to teach and assess student learning. You see by trade I am a nurse practitioner and until my doctoral program, never had any formal training on how to educate, what curriculum meant, and what in the world the American Association of Colleges of Nursing (AACN) was. I simply found a passion to share knowledge with others and that bloomed into the nursing education career that I am experiencing today. As I write this text, I am thinking of those who have come before me as well as those who are following behind. I am keenly aware of my place in this spectrum, and feel privileged that you, a fellow nurse educator or nursing student, would choose to read about my ideas.

This text was written for those who have no idea what the flipped classroom is but are intrigued and for those who have a good idea what the flipped classroom is and are looking for some guidance. My work with the flipped classroom has been a true adventure, full of valuable experiential learning. I tend to jump into a new idea about teaching and learning with both feet regardless of the warning signs. Okay, I admit, I didn't even look for any warning signs before I jumped on this one. I saw such an exciting potential for this method that I just went with it. But I believe that this blind leap of faith was for a purpose. I learned so much from my experiences in flipping trial and error that helped me to form ideas about the flipped classroom and how it can be implemented specifically within nursing education. I made many mistakes that have all helped me to learn the right and not so right ways to implement the flipped classroom in nursing education. So it is my goal for you to learn from my mistakes and gain this knowledge for yourselves in an easier manner.

Once I took time to find texts and information about the flipped classroom, it was clear to me that this was *a* teaching and learning method explored primarily in the K-12 classrooms. Although there are many of us out there flipping our nursing classrooms, there are not many publications, research articles, or self-help guides to make the process an easier one. I hope you will find this text to be extremely timely and useful to your nursing education classroom and to your students. I have had the privilege to work with some pioneers of flipping who have taught me many more strategies and "secrets" of the trade so to speak. The compilation of knowledge about the flipped classroom within nursing education and the lack of higher education textbooks to help instructors attempt to flip were the impetus for this book.

Throughout my many nursing education experiences, it was not uncommon to find myself in a classroom with a lecturing instructor performing monotonous PowerPoint karaoke. Perhaps you can relate to the scene. As the lecturer discussed the finer points of acid-base balance, I attempted to furiously take notes and simultaneously listen to the lecture. Just as I would get done writing down one point, I would miss the next important point about the process that was being relayed by my instructor. I always seemed to be too busy writing to really listen. Somewhere around slide 47, I began to realize that I didn't understand one or more parts of the intricate acid-base balance that would be occurring within my soon-to-be patient's body. Instead of stopping the instructor, I allowed the lecture to continue on with additional content building upon that which I did not understand. I didn't ask a question for fear of being identified as "that person" in the class who wasn't getting it. Sometimes I was so lost I didn't even know what question I should ask to help my confusion. Frustrated, I would go home to read and re-read the chapter or try to reach out to my peers who might be able to help me understand the content. Most of the time this was a disappointing venture, because I would soon find out that they didn't really get it either.

Because most nursing instructors have been educated through these types of lectures, it is not uncommon for them to teach the way in which they were taught. Even though I consider myself to be a fairly entertaining lecturer, I have those moments when I am watching the students in my classroom slowly fade into a coma as I attempt to dazzle them with the best of my lecturing ability. I have often wondered when my aptitude to entertain a crowd became such an integral part of my teaching regimen. I have been a nurse educator for quite some time and have talked to many fellow nurse educators. In my conversations with other nurse educators, it has been confirmed that many have had similar experiences with lecture in their own classrooms. It would be safe to say that the majority of educators might agree that even the most engaging of lecturer has noticed the occasional yawn, spaced-out face, or ever-texting student in the crowd.

It is understandable why students might lose attention during any lecture. They are, after all, human. Most of us know that the average attention span of an adult learner has been estimated at around 8 seconds, down from 12 seconds less than a decade ago (Statistic Brain Research Institute, 2015). Some experts believe that the increasing external stimulation of the human brain from various mobile devices, stimulating video games, and flashy Internet websites may be to blame for the decreased attention span of today's students. In the last 18 years that I have been in the nursing education classroom, I have noticed more and more of these types of digital devices, laptop computers, tablets, digital phones, and the like on the desks of my students. At times I find myself wondering if these students are really paying attention to the class or busy updating their Facebook accounts.

I do remember a student several years ago shout out during class with joy as she was able to obtain tickets to the Colorado Rockies baseball playoff game. This was indeed a shocker for me as her instructor, because she had been so diligently watching the screen of her computer in what I had assumed was her concentration on the PowerPoint slides I had provided prior to class. It was not however a surprise to those around her, who had seen the other side of that screen all along. They of course shared in her joy while she interrupted my lecture and class to describe just how close she would be to the baseline. Unfortunately, this is the type of technology multitasking that students are engaged with in our classes. This student quickly explained to me that there was no disrespect to me as an instructor, but it was after all the playoffs. I did not share in her joy or accept her explanation for why she was physically but obviously not mentally present in class that day. Needless to say we had a little talk after class and she assured me it would not happen again . . . until next baseball season?

This example is just one of the many stories to describe and helps to explain how many of our students are not above "multitasking" in the classroom, which is a facade all in its own. Researchers such as Earl Miller, a Picower professor of neuroscience at Massachusetts Institute of Technology (MIT), continue to report that multitasking is a myth, regardless of the current technology that allows people to believe in the notion (Hamilton, 2008). Humans cannot do more than one task at a time, but are efficient at switching attention from one task to another very quickly. This ability fools us into thinking that we are "multitasking," when really we are splitting our attention quickly, only mentally present for seconds at a time. We may think we are doing more things and in fact may get more things completed, but are we doing things correctly or to the utmost of our ability? This is another question altogether.

How Are the Students of Today Unique?

There are some authors that do not believe that students are hindered at all by their attention span, but by the style of teaching within the classroom. They argue that students who have a difficult time sitting still or paying attention in a classroom might be the same students who can sit for hours in front of a video game or movie that they find interesting. Mark Prensky (2010) poses some important differences about students of today in his text about teaching digital natives. This group of student has learned to focus on what interests them and on things that make them feel like an individual versus part of a group. He posits that in the increasingly populated world with multiple choices at the fingertips, the need for differentiation, personalization, and individualization have become a necessity in the young people of today. If we think about the world that these students are living within, it is filled with opportunities on social media to "create" their own digital identities and footprint on the social media landscape. The term "digital branding" or "personal branding" describes how students are creating a digital identity for themselves. There are some very popular websites that were created for this type of individualization, creating a chance to show everyone else in the world who they are and what they are thinking, doing, and feeling at any given moment. This group is called ***"digital natives."***

Palfrey and Gasser (2008) define *digital natives* as those born after 1980, when digital technologies, social media, and Web-based informational systems were already in full swing. Major aspects of the digital native's life, such as social interactions, friendships, and information gathering, are mediated by social digital technologies. The digital native has never known any other environment, but to date there has not been a generation that has lived from birth to death within the digital era (2008). By contrast, many faculty are considered "digital immigrants." *Digital immigrants* are those who remember a world before the widespread use of the home personal computers, the World Wide Web, various forms of social media, and handheld devices. Most faculty and others born before 1980, never even owned a cell phone until the mid-1990s whereas children now as young as 5 years old are accessing handheld devices on long trips in the car with their parents thinking how blessed their children are to have that kind of technology at their fingertips. Parents are raising little digital natives who know how to run some of the Internet sites and programs better than their parents do. It is incredible that children are growing up with the ability to "google" any subject and find the answer. By contrast, digital immigrants had to dig through dusty encyclopedias that were 10 years out of date and sometimes never found the answer to their questions, even in a well-stocked library. Digital immigrants used to write letters to one another and wait weeks for a response, had only three channels of television with wavy lines through each picture, and met people at the ice cream shop, park, or at a school dance rather than finding one another on Facebook or some other digitally created society. Digital immigrants only learned to email and search the Internet when they were already nursing professionals, or at least when they were in school. And yes, some nursing professionals learned how to type on an old electric typewriter with keys and corrective fluid! Kids today don't know how lucky they are to have the delete button and spell checker on the computer. Nursing professionals have the vast knowledge about the profession that they can share with the next generation and are in a prime position to use this digital world to their advantage. But how do we go about teaching this digital native student community effectively? What do these digital natives want to see within their educational experience? Prensky (2010) has conducted almost a thousand interviews with digital native students and has found the following to be true:

1. They do not want to be lectured to.
2. They want to be respected and trusted, and to have their own opinions and have those opinions be heard, valued, and for them to count.
3. They want to follow their own interests and passions.
4. They want to create using the tools of their time (including the digital tools).

5. They want to work with their peers, share ideas, and be a part of group work and projects, but also want to prevent slackers from getting a "free ride."
6. They want to make decisions and at least share control.
7. They want to be able to connect with their peers, share their opinions not only in your class but also with the world.
8. They want to not only cooperate with one another, but also compete against each other.
9. They want an education that is not only relevant, but also real (Prensky, 2010, pp. 2–3).

Although this list seems like narcissistic expectations with which Prensky agrees, he also believes that continuing on with this as the main thought is a mistake of educators. Instead, educators need to think of these expectations as a change of the times and reflective of the fact that students want to learn differently today, because they live in a digital world. Students want to learn from educators, but they also want their education to be immediately relevant to their role within society, their profession, and the world. This forward thinking of the digital native students puts them in a global mindset that nursing educators can really take advantage of.

Even though the digital native seems to be a bit spoiled by their self-serving digital world, consider some of the additional challenges that they may be facing while in nursing school. For example, the average nursing student is more likely to be dealing with additional social and financial challenges than students in the past. The twenty-first century student obtains less sleep on average (University of Georgia, 2015) and a financial condition that may require them to be employed while in college, in some cases close to full-time employment (CBS News, 2013). Many students are returning for a degree after they begin their families as well. The added domestic tasks of the average student, coupled with sleep deprivation and the need to work while in school leaves little time for studying.

I had an interesting conversation with a group of students in the hallway one day. Being in their major medical-surgical nursing course, I asked them how they were getting through the large amount of reading that they undoubtedly had been doing. They reported that they really liked their course and felt like their professor was very knowledgeable, which did not surprise me. What did surprise me was their comment about not having to buy the textbook. Of course this piqued my interest as an instructor, because I assumed all students not only purchased the textbook, but at least attempted to read every page I had recommended for their learning. After further probing, these students reported that they had a required textbook clearly listed in the syllabus, but their instructor told them everything that they needed to know in lecture anyway, so why buy the book or read it for that matter? The students noted that they could just search on the Internet for a Web-based video on the topic instead of reading about it in the expensive, oversized required textbook. The students did not see anything abnormal about this approach at all, a stark contrast to my viewpoint. This was just their reality and current learning culture. I soon realized that *I* was the one with the outdated expectations. I had "grown up" in a different educational time than these students, and came to recognize that my expectations were coming from my past education, not the current state of our digital world. Now don't get me wrong, I still have a required textbook and plenty of required readings. But now my class is not filled with lectures where I basically tell them everything that they should have read in the textbook anyway. Instead, they are asked to do their readings and then watch a short highlights or clinical pearls video I create for them that augments their reading at home. Once they get to my classroom, they are ready to apply the information they have read and learned from their readings and the videos at home.

How Can Flipped Learning Be Effective in Nursing Education?

Nurse educators are up against some major barriers as they teach this digitally intelligent and stimulated population. Although the healthcare system and nursing in general have undergone some major revisions, many of the educational classrooms have not followed suit. This book is about a teaching method called *flipped learning* or the *flipped classroom* that has the potential to change teaching and learning for nursing education. We can teach in a way that reflects the changing landscape of nursing education and the technologically savvy students within. Although there appears to be no "educational utopia," we do have the power as individual educators to transform our classrooms with the goal of maximizing the best learning outcomes for our over-stressed and over-stimulated students.

Remember the scenario in the acid-base balance lecture at the beginning of the chapter? Think for a moment how much different that educational interchange might have been if each student could have watched the lecture at home on their personal computer or other device prior to coming to class? Each student would have had the ability to stop and restart the video or rewind to areas that they didn't understand. Each student would have been able to take notes on what the professor had said during the video because they were able to pause the video at the specific point of misunderstanding. Imagine the potential for individual learning if each student could search for the answer to their own question as they put the lecture on hold. My students have often told me that I talk too fast in my lectures. I jokingly tell them that they need to think faster to keep up with me. But truly they have a point here. Depending on the students in the classroom, I think about 80% of them keep pace with the lecture and my pace of speech. What happens to the other 20%? Now imagine that all of the students who had a hard time keeping up with my lecture can now not only "pause" me to write things down, but could also slow my speech down to a desirable level. This idea really resonated with me, because students have the power that they need to move through the lecture material at their own pace. Those who kept pace also have the opportunity to view and review again the lecture to help solidify their understanding. If they want, they can even speed up the video to save them some time (as long as I am *nowhere* near to hear the faster more high-pitched mouse-like version of my voice in this mode!). The point is, the students have my lecture at their fingertips and can move through it at their own pace. They can take notes at their own speed, and more importantly, take the time to write down their questions and bring them to class. In the classroom setting, each student's questions are addressed individually as part of the flipped classroom model.

Before I started to use the flipped classroom, I would use quite a bit of Socratic Method to attempt to engage the students while in lecture. Of course, I noticed that most of the time, the same 4 or 5 students answered all of my questions. So I started writing every student's on my roster down on a 3 × 5 card at the beginning of the semester. I would shuffle them at the beginning of class and then pick names randomly from the top of the "deck." I still do this within my flipped classroom because it insures that each student is getting a chance to participate in a discussion. It was when I started this method of randomization of student engagement in the classroom that I noted some glaring cultural differences in my students. Some of the cultural backgrounds of students would lend them to being more quiet and shy, while other cultures did not mind at all talking or even shouting over one another to get into the mix of the discussion. I have noticed that when using the flipped classroom, students from various cultures feel more comfortable sharing their ideas, particularly one on one and in smaller groups. Part of the classroom strategies I will discuss in this text will show more of how to engage students of varying cultures into the mainstream discussion and class activities.

So What Exactly Is Flipped Learning?

Over the past several decades, nursing educators have attempted many different and innovative teaching and learning techniques. Providing a learning environment that is more active than passive has been gaining popularity in many nursing classrooms, and in most cases the benefits to nursing students seem to outweigh the extra planning and class preparation time of the faculty. Many of these so-called "active learning" strategies, problem-based learning, cooperative learning and the like, have changed the way nursing content is delivered in many programs and classrooms across the nation. So what is the big deal about flipped learning or the flipped classroom?

How is flipped learning any different than what is already being done within the nursing classroom? Largely the answer lies in the burst of technology over the last several years. Within this surge in technology, the ability to record lectures and provide them in easily accessible ways to students is one of the key factors in the flipped learning model. The Flipped Classroom is a term coined by two high school chemistry teachers, Jonathan Bergmann and Aaron Sams (2012). Dealing with catching students up after excused absences, these two innovators learned about "lecture capture software" that would record a lecture on the computer screen (screen capture) with the instructors talking students through slides in a compact recording. These recorded lectures were made available to the students online to view at their convenience. Seeing the potential for more meaningful interaction time with students in the classroom, they decided to "flip" the traditional homework time with the traditional in-class lecture time. In this new "flipped classroom," the students watched a recorded lecture originally delivered during the in-class time and used class time to work through problems and homework to apply that material while their teachers were present (**Figure 1-1**). The ability to use screen capture software and launch it online to a student audience made this type of teaching and learning atmosphere possible.

Along with the original definition of the flipped classroom or flipped learning already reviewed, an official definition has been developed by the experts at the Flipped Learning Network.

Flipped Learning is defined as a pedagogical approach in which direct instruction moves from the group learning space to the individual learning space, and the resulting group space is transformed into a dynamic, interactive learning environment where the educator guides the students as they apply concepts and engage creatively in the subject matter (The Flipped Learning Network, 2014).

TRADITIONAL CLASSROOM

- Students do readings at home and print out PowerPoint notes for lecture
- Instructor prepares lecture materials
- Students listen to lecture by instructor
- Students take notes on the lecture
- The instructor is the center of the class
- The instructor is in control of class time

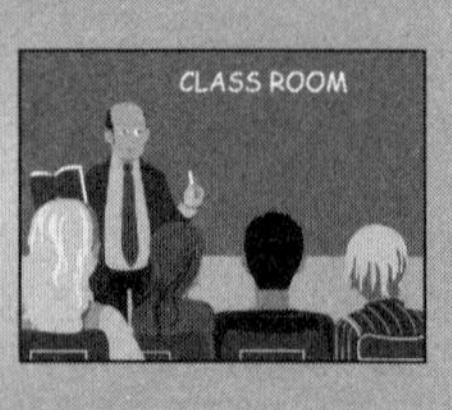

FLIPPED CLASSROOM

Lecture at Home:

- Instructor prepares lecture and delivers to students prior to class via video
- *Class is focused on student application of what they learned on the video with many group and some individual activities*
- Instructor is able to support students and assess individual learning
- *Students are at the center of the class*

Figure 1-1 What does it look like?

Notice that the definition does not mention anything about video capture of lectures. The main idea behind the flipped learning model is to *maximize the time the students and faculty have during the face-to-face* time in the classroom. The flipped model is not about delivering course content online only, students working without any structure, working in isolation or spending their entire class time at a computer screen. The flipped model is an opportunity for increased contact time between faculty and students engaging the application of course content rather than lecture format where material is delivered to students by the instructor. The model requires that students take responsibility for their own learning in a classroom learning environment that involves application of rote information and engagement of each and every student in the classroom. This class description fits perfectly with nursing education due to the need for students to be able to critically think through patient symptoms and interventions within short periods of time. Please see **Table 1-1** for a comparison of the flipped model and traditional lecture teaching methods.

Table 1-1 Comparison of Traditional and Flipped Classrooms

	Traditional Classroom	Flipped Classroom
Definition	Traditional teaching is concerned with the teacher being the controller of the learning environment. Power and responsibility are held by the teacher and teachers play the role of instructor (in the form of lectures) and decision maker. They regard students as having "knowledge holes" that need to be filled with information. In short, the traditional teacher views that it is the teacher that causes learning to occur.	Flipped learning is defined as a pedagogical approach in which direct instruction moves from the group learning space to the individual learning space, and the resulting group space is transformed into a dynamic, interactive learning environment where the educator guides the students as they apply concepts and engage creatively in the subject matter.
Context	The instructor provides a lecture, perhaps intertwined with Socratic method type questioning, providing a "sage on the stage" atmosphere. The instructor is the main conduit of knowledge delivering content to the students.	The instructor's lecture is captured with technology and provided to the students prior to class. In class the instructor becomes the "guide on the side," helping the students with common questions and application of the materials.
Philosophy	The instructor causes learning to occur in the form of lecture and audiovisuals.	The students learn by active methods and application.
Tools	PowerPoints with slides of material to cover, notes for students to follow, perhaps use of video	Lecture capture loaded on Web or learning management system, high-speed Internet access, tools for engaging learning activities during classroom time allowed
Assignments	Readings, reviewing notes of lecture slides	Readings and viewing lectures prior to class Assignments vary depending on methods used in classroom and methods of evaluation employed.

(*Continues*)

Table 1-1 Comparison of Traditional and Flipped Classrooms (Continued)

	Traditional Classroom	Flipped Classroom
Advantages	Instructor able to deliver content that is important and necessary to cover during classroom time. Students are used to this type of educational environment for the most part. Easy to lecture and deliver information to students.	Allows students to be more engaged in their own learning. Allows for different learning styles and cultures to be accommodated. Forces students to be engaged and active learners in the classroom. Allows for the instructor to answer questions and correct errors in thinking that may go unnoticed in a traditional classroom. Ability to use technology that digital students are comfortable with. Uses time effectively for full content delivery.
Limitations	Puts learner in an inactive role. Time limitations to provide active learning activities.	Requires an understanding of technology and how to use. Students resistant to method at first. Faculty need to spend more time to prepare when lecture materials may be already done.
Challenges	May not actively engage learners. Allows students to be passive in the teaching/learning environment.	Difficult to change culture of learning once already established. Technology can be difficult to use and does not always work the way it should. Takes a significant amount of preparation time.

Although the term and associated concepts of the "flipped classroom" are new, the active teaching and learning are not. It is not uncommon for nursing faculty to provide a teaching/learning environment that requires the student to actively learn the material and apply it to real-life scenarios. Some other terms that have been used to describe an active or more student-engaged learning environment include blended learning, collaborative learning, and active learning. When viewed through the lens of the educator who has been involved in this type of classroom for years, the flipped classroom model may appear to be an old strategy with a new name. However, those who have done in-depth reading and research on the flipped classroom recognize several key differences inherent in the model. One possible reason for the excitement attached to the term "flipped classroom" comes from the addition of technological advances to the application of the teaching/learning process. In a way, the educator can have their cake and eat it too.

One of the main barriers to providing a more active learning environment for many educators has been the increasing amount of material that needs to be covered coupled with the shrinking amount of face-to-face time with the students in the classroom. There never seems to be enough time in a 2- or 3-hour class period to both deliver a lecture about important concepts and also engage students in active learning. I have always invited students to ask questions in the classroom during lectures, but have found that doing so at times took time away from the other students' learning atmosphere who had different questions. Similarly, those who understood everything were left idle during the time it took to explain the concept and answer an individual student question. As you know, this is just an open invitation for students to disengage and move on to other tasks, particularly with digital devices in the classroom, happy to assist with their "mind vacation."

With the flipped model, I have found time to address individual questions from my students with a small group instruction design. As an instructor, I am able to get to every student's questions about the material that they have he or she has viewed ahead of time in the pre-class video. In a way, this allows the "mastery" learning that Bergmann and Sams (2012) have discussed in their flipped learning publications. Although in nursing we tend to keep every student on the same subject for each class, I have found that with the flipped model, I am able to address individual learning needs and allow students to move on with other content once they have mastered the objectives of the unit. Of course, the mastery model takes quite a bit of preparation on my part as the instructor, but it is not as bad as one might think. I simply plan for those students who are grasping concepts more easily to move on to more complex issues. I have done this by preparing several case studies of increasing difficulty. I will admit I am new at the mastery model, but I am finding that it does allow more accommodation for different learning paces that we often see in a group of students within the classroom.

How Can I Flip My Hybrid Course?

We have discussed what the flipped classroom looks like in the typically face-to-face classroom we are accustomed to, but what about other forms of course delivery? Hybrid course delivery is defined differently by each institution, but a general definition includes blending some in-class time with online class time. What differs per institution is the amount of the course that should be online within a hybrid, versus totally online, versus totally in-class time frame. Most universities allow for somewhere around 20% of a face-to-face to be online, but around 40% to 50% of the course within a hybrid course, and of course an online course is in most cases 100% online. Some individual definitions from specific universities may be helpful, for these see **Table 1-2**.

Conducting the flipped model in the blended or hybrid format should make quite a bit of sense. Instructional designers are experts at developing a course and its related objectives around any type of format. It would be my first suggestion to take advantage of any of these experts that may be available to you in your area. Their expertise can help you in planning your hybrid course and implementing the flipped model within. In general, the online portion of the course lends itself well to implementation of the video lecture material. Along with the assignment of the video lecture, it would be my advice to assign some sort of evaluation method to accompany the video lecture. The easiest of these assignments or learning assessments, in my opinion, is an online quiz. There are some faculty who

Table 1-2 Definitions of Hybrid Course Format

Oregon State University (OSU)	"A hybrid course blends online components and required face-to-face class meetings. A substantial portion of the learning activities are delivered online . . . face-to-face meeting time is reduced by 40% compared to traditional on-campus course" OSU (2015).
The George Washington University	"A hybrid approach to education (also known as 'blended'), whether in a single course or threaded throughout a program, balances face-to-face and online environments. A course is generally considered hybrid when the percentage of work done online is between 30–70%" (The George Washington University, 2015).
Northern Virginia Community College (NOVA)	"Typically, your hybrid course will meet 50 percent of the time in the classroom and 50 percent online" (NOVA, 2015).
West LA College	"A hybrid class combines classroom learning with online learning. In a hybrid course, a significant portion of the class learning activities are online, which reduces the amount of time spent in a traditional, face-to-face classroom" (West LA College, 2015).

are adamant about not providing online quizzes, knowing that the students will use resources and not be observed by faculty. Of course, this provides a perfect environment for cheating. I used to share this viewpoint as well. But now I have come to realize that if students are accessing their resources, they are just emulating the same type of activity I want them to as practicing nurses. I want them to be able to understand what resources to use and how to access them. To that end, part of the learning assessment in an open-book, open-note online quiz is finding the correct resources in a reasonable amount of time, and applying that information to find out the answer to a question. This is not unlike the fast-paced clinical environment the students will be working in as nursing professionals.

Other online learning assessments to assign in the online portion of a hybrid course might be assignment sheets directly related to the video lectures, group discussions, small group, and other assignments that involve engagement with additional resources or the community.

For example, in a hybrid community health course, one might have a unit about community resources that stretches over both online and in class-time periods. Depending on the type of objectives written for this section, it would be helpful to do a lecture video on community resources, and the importance of a nurse understanding community resources for referral to serve a variety of patient populations. Split the class into small groups, each with a different assignment related to community resources. For example, one group would be assigned resources related to poverty, another would be assigned resources for the psychiatric population, another group would look at resources for women, another for children, another for the elderly, another for the immigrant population, and so on. For the online portion of the course, the student would watch the lecture video and then have an assignment related to seeking out the resources for their assigned group. Of course, a formal set of goals or objectives for the assignment and a rubric to help guide students in the assignment would be helpful. I always try to put in the assignment some kind of engagement with the community resource, like a short interview with a central employee at one of the resources the student has found. Most community agencies are very willing to help with these types of assignments, particularly when I contact them ahead of time and let them know that the students may be requesting a few minutes of their time.

When the class meets for face-to-face time, each student will be asked to bring their assignment and share the community resources they learned about. Let's say that there were 36 students in the class and 6 groups of 6 students looked at similar resources. A jigsaw is a helpful in-class teaching/learning strategy in which one student from each group is reassigned into a group that contains one student from each of the other groups. The newly formed groups, each with a student that reviewed and accessed different community resources, is assigned the task of creating a "community resource guide" that can be then be distributed to the rest of the class. The jigsaw is one of my favorite activities, but it is difficult to explain in narrative form. For more on this type of interactive teaching/learning method, please see the In-Class Activities chapter.

How Can I Flip My Online Course?

The online course environment is not directly conducive to the flipped learning model, because the flipped classroom as it is defined is focused on maximizing the face-to-face time between faculty member and student. Online courses do not typically have any face-to-face time with the instructor, so this produces a bit of a challenge. There are some instructors that are using a modified version of flipping within the online environment. The video lecture material is delivered in the same way as in the traditional flipped or hybrid formats. The instructor sets up "virtual office hours" 2 or 3 times a week. During these office hours, the instructor opens some type of digital, virtual classroom environment where the students are encouraged to access the instructor, ask questions, and complete other assignments. Within most learning management systems, there is an online video chat available. To really make this type of online classroom flipped, the students need to commit to one of the times available in order to engage with the faculty member as part of their coursework. Many students choose online courses due to their asynchronous nature and freedom from any specified class times they need to be present during the course. Requiring any face-to-face time in a course designed and advertised in the course catalogue as totally online may cause some problems regarding student expectations of the course. If this type of flipping online format would be used, it would be highly recommended that it is listed as such within the course syllabus and course catalogue, and that students receive some sort of percentage of their course grade for being "virtually present" in these predetermined class times.

Flipped Learning—Can It Address the Current Challenges of Nursing Education?

It is probably obvious to even the most novice of nurse educators that prelicensure nursing curricula are bulging at the seams with content that needs to be covered for basic entry into practice knowledge. The American Association of Colleges of Nursing (AACN) Essentials for Nursing Education have provided curricular suggestions for undergraduate and graduate programs of nursing for decades. These essentials for college and university education for professional nursing were first published in 1986, with revisions in 1998 and 2008 (AACN, 2015). Each revision has provided more detailed and complex content for nursing curricula to cover at both the graduate and undergraduate levels. With so many topics and multifaceted issues for nurses to learn on top of the crucial skill performance in clinical settings, it is becoming more and more difficult for nurse educators to meet the essentials set forth by the AACN for nursing education. This text suggests that nurse educators take advantage of the stair-step learning opportunities of Bloom's taxonomy (Bloom, Engelhart, Furst, Hill, & Krathwohl, 1956) to help with this dilemma.

What's Bloom's Got to Do With It?

Most, if not all, educators are familiar with Bloom's taxonomy. The taxonomy is a classification system of the different objectives that educators set for student learning within a course or program. So where did Bloom's taxonomy come from? The idea of a classification system for student learning was formed at an informal meeting of college professors attending an American Psychology Association Convention in Boston in 1948. This group of experts lead by Benjamin Bloom, an American educational psychologist from the University of Chicago, was interested in a theoretical framework that could be used to facilitate communication among examiners and promote the exchange of test materials and ideas about testing. It was also thought that such a framework could stimulate research examining the relationship between exams and education. The discussion led to a realization that a system classifying the goals of the educational process would be the natural basis for the framework as they are used to build curricula and shape the associated student outcome assessments (Bloom et al., 1956). The committee met yearly and developed the first iteration of what is known as Bloom's taxonomy. Within the original taxonomy were three domains: cognitive, affective, and psychomotor. In the 1990s a former student of

Bloom's, Lorin Anderson, led a new group of cognitive psychologists in the updating of the original taxonomy.

Bloom's taxonomy assumes that within the three domains of cognitive, affective, and psychomotor, learning at higher levels is dependent on having obtained prerequisite knowledge and skills at lower levels. The photo depiction (**Figure 1-2**) of the original taxonomy indicates that students must master content first by remembering, then by understanding, followed by applying that information, and then finally being able to use that information for analysis, evaluation, and creation of new knowledge.

It could be argued that using only lecture during the face-to-face time available in the nursing education classroom engages the student at the lowest level of Bloom's taxonomy. What if we could engage the student with lecture material at these lower levels of the

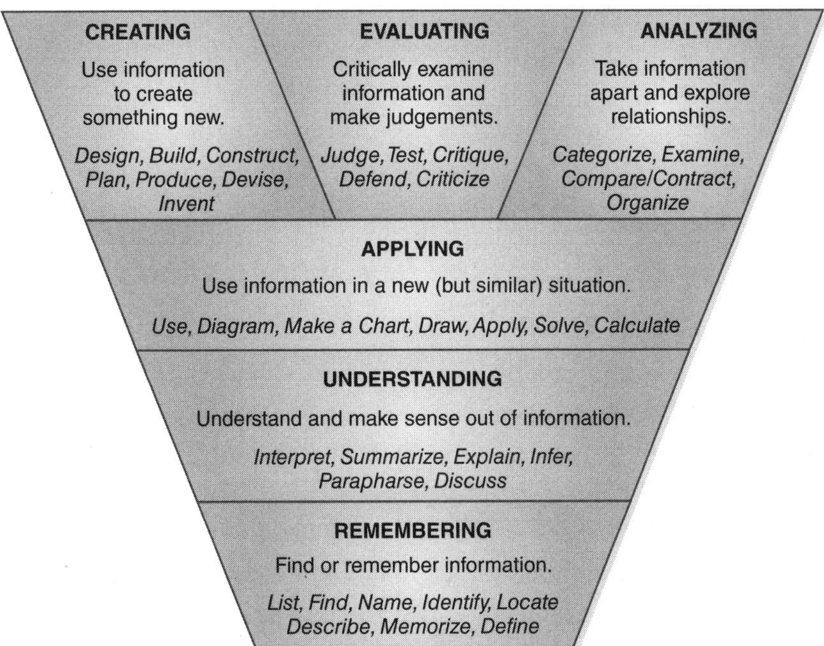

Figure 1-2 Bloom's taxonomy.

taxonomy prior to them coming to our face-to-face classroom? How much farther could we move up the Bloom's taxonomy ladder if we had students apply their knowledge and understanding of content with the instructor there to help them do so? Would it be possible to then teach at a higher level of the taxonomy every time we have face-to-face classes? It seems that this would be entirely possible and not only that, very feasible. By providing any rote memorization and lower levels of remembering and understanding through lectures at home prior to coming to face-to-face classes, students would be ready to apply the material and move toward analysis and the critical thinking realm that educators desire of their students.

In the flipped classroom model, the educator is still able to provide a lecture that is recorded and provided to the student online. When the students come to class (in the best-case scenario), they have already heard the lecture that the educator would have normally delivered in the face-to-face classroom. The preview of lecture material opens up the scheduled classroom time for more engaging teaching/learning activities with the nurse educator as the guide on the side. The time spent on lecture-type material is replaced with time to help each student or group of students apply the material, ask questions about how the concepts can be applied to a patient case scenario, and provide a more active way to learn.

Flipping the Classroom in Light of the IOM Report and Benner's Latest Work

In the most recent Institute of Medicine (IOM, 2011) report on the future of nursing and nursing education, nursing education and practice experts from across the nation gathered their expertise to address the most important issues in the profession to date. The experts published suggestions on "how to teach" nurses include guiding students in the integration of knowledge from the clinical, social, and behavioral sciences with the practice of nursing in order to enhance development of critical thinking skills. Also included in the recommendations was development of a curriculum that supported best practices in teaching and learning.

The most recent text by Finkelman and Kenner (2012) focused on how nurse educators should implement the IOM recommendations to prepare the next generation of nurses. Within the main summary points from the February 2010 Forum on *The Future of Nursing Education* are many areas where use of the flipped classroom has the potential to address key issues found within our existing educational system. **Table 1-3** provides a few of these content items along with how the flipped classroom has the potential to address or at the very least assist with integration of the recommendations. The flipped learning model has the potential to help nurse educators implement these IOM recommendations in a meaningful way using something as simple as a new teaching and learning strategy.

Benner, Sutphen, Leonard, and Day's (2010) work echo many of the same suggestions as Finkelman and Kenner (2012) on how to transform nursing education. Benner and colleagues' work with the Carnegie Foundation for the Advancement of Teaching culminated in a national study focusing on nursing education and a text titled, *Educating Nurses: A Call for Radical Transformation.* The goal of the study the book was founded upon was to understand how nurse educators were preparing students to enter the profession. This work is just phenomenal, and provides a framework for change within the way we educate nurses. These authors posit that "a significant gap exists between today's nursing practice and the education for that practice, despite some considerable strengths in nursing education" (2010, p. 4). Adding more and more to each curriculum will not be sufficient, because the quality of what and how we teach must be at a higher level to meet the challenges of the changing healthcare landscape of the nation. Even if there were no nursing shortage and no shortage of nursing faculty, nursing education would still be in need of dramatic change to meet the demands of current nursing practice (2010).

Table 1-3 IOM Forum on the Future of Nursing Education and Flipped Learning

The Future of Nursing Recommendation	How Can Flipped Learning Address the Recommendation?
"The new basics in nursing education include collaboration within the profession and across other health professions, communication, and systems thinking" (Finkelman & Kenner, 2012, p. 37).	Several of the in-class activities students will engage in within the flipped model can help foster communication and systems thinking. Although this is not different than other collaborative learning styles of learning, it does provide more time for these types of activities.
Nurses, particularly nurse educators, need to keep up with a rapidly changing knowledge base and new technologies throughout their careers to ensure a well-educated workforce.	The key term in this recommendation is new technology. If we can master the current technology and help our students to do the same (or maybe vise versa), flipped learning will augment knowledge base about how to adapt to new technologies of a similar nature.
Technology that fosters problem-solving and critical thinking skills in nurses is essential for nursing education to produce sufficient numbers of competent, well-educated nurses.	Even though this recommendation is focused somewhat on high-fidelity simulation, it also speaks to the need for more problem-solving and critical thinking skills. Within the flipped classroom, students engage at a higher level of learning taxonomy and are able to work on critical thinking and problemsolving both individually and in groups. These environments foster not only knowledge building, but also a safe environment where there exists not only time for questions related to content, the class is structured around remaining questions and finding those answers.
In addition to necessary skill sets, nursing education should provide students with the ability to mature as professionals and to continue learning throughout their careers.	One aspect of flipped learning that I am excited about, is the potential to create a "spirit of inquiry" for each and every student in the classroom. In the evidence-based world we now live within in nursing, we no longer just listen to someone tell us what we need to know. Instead, we are knowledge seekers. We go out and find what we need to know to safely care for our patients at the highest levels of quality. If we can teach our students to do this every day or every week in the classroom and the clinical settings, we could come a long way in the development of a generation of life-long learners.

Benner et al. (2010) have discussed the "theory" portion of the nursing classroom, which is referred to by the authors as "a range of substantive knowledge about nursing care, nursing theory, nursing science, biology, chemistry, and physics, and medical interventions that nurses need to master" (p. 13). During their research, the authors observed several nursing education classrooms and clinical learning experiences. While observing the "theory" classrooms (what others may consider didactic) they describe a learning environment in sharp contrast to the skillful and effective teaching approaches witnessed within clinical settings. First of all, the material was typically presented in a highly abstract way, with lectures that appeared to be standardized and delivered through slide presentations. The students were presented information about the physiology, disease categories, signs and symptoms, interventions, and outcomes to be memorized. The "presentation" word seems to stick out within this scenario. It was the authors' observation, one that was reinforced by faculty and students, that widespread reliance on slide presentation and standardized lectures was the norm within the classroom time provided. I love the scene these authors set—may I share it with you?

In our site visits we saw many classes begin with students opening their notebooks to an outline of the lecture and ending with the teacher at the front of the room having shown the last of dozens of slides. As the teacher glided from slide to slide, the students made notes in the margins of their course outlines, collectively turning their pages at every sixth slide. Discussion was cursory and some faculty even limited questions, not wanting to be pulled too far from the slide presentation (Benner et al., 2010, p. 13).

Although this way of teaching may seem tempting as a way to compress the bigger and bigger curriculum topics into the time allotted within the classroom, it is actually defies the way in which we learn. It also discourages the type of learning or environment that fosters the way a nurse must use knowledge as they think in ever-changing clinical situations, a necessary skill for successful nursing practice. Nursing is a practice discipline that relies on situation cognition and actions (Benner et al., 2010). If teaching occurs as in the scenario of lecture above, students are learning about patient care in segmented chunks. My colleague, Katherine (Kat) Johnson, and I came to this realization within one of the family nurse practitioner (FNP) courses we taught together. We were using lecture as our main teaching strategy, with a little bit of Socratic method thrown in to keep everyone awake and alert (including ourselves). We were looking over one of the student exams together and began to realize that we were testing them using patient care scenarios. So really we were leaving a large portion of our job as educators up to the students to grapple with on their own time and without any guidance and/or assistance from us as their instructors. The proverbial light came on for us at that moment. We realized that we were not providing them the practice and application of the material in order for them to be successful on their exams and in the clinical settings. We were teaching them silos of information in class, and then expecting them to somehow miraculously put it all together expertly within a simulated clinical situation on their exams.

Similarly, Benner et al. (2010) found in their study what they described as "a tenacious assumption that the student learns abstract information and then *applies* that information in practice" (p. 14). They've suggested that learning complex and evolving information to apply in the high-stakes environment of nursing practice calls for "an ongoing dialogue between information and practice, between the particular and the general, so that students build an evidence base for care and thus learn to make decisions about appropriate interventions for the particular patient" (p. 14). If the students can build this knowledge base to apply to any patient care situation, they have come a long way in the journey of recognizing the critical, most urgent aspects of each individual patient they care for.

We can apply what we've learned from Benner's (2001) Novice to Expert work and from our knowledge of Cognitive Load Theory to our teaching within the classroom. Both theories focus on the fact that for learning to occur, the human brain must be able to practice, practice, and practice again. I am sure Benner is aware, but the cognitive load theory fits very nicely with her work in applying the Dreyfus model of skill acquisition to the nursing profession. The more practice and exposure students have to different types of scenarios using the same basic information, the more expert their brain becomes at storing information into the long-term memory. That information can then be quickly recalled to short-term memory whenever it is needed. In the nursing education classroom, it is not uncommon for us to "present" a large amount of information using lectures and expect each student to absorb, understand, analyze, and then apply it to clinical situations. I think it is worth the time to take a closer look at Cognitive Load Theory.

Cognitive Load Theory (CLT) was first discussed by John Swellar and colleagues, who suggested that learning occurred best in an environment that appreciates the student's existing human cognitive architecture (Swellar, van Merrienboer, & Paas, 1998). The theory can be applied to how we design the way in which we teach students in complex and technically challenging professions such as nursing. According to CLT, instructors must have a solid understanding of how students are processing and storing data in the brain during any pedagogical event. Memory consists of both short-term and long-term memory (Atkinson & Shiffrin, 1968). According to CLT, learning occurs when there is accumulation of knowledge and addition to information within the long-term memory (Swellar et al., 1998). When a student begins to process new information, he/she does so first within the short-term memory, which contains sensory and working memory. Sensory memory is limited to about 20 seconds of attention capacity and allows for filtering of pieces of information as either relevant or non-relevant (Atkinson & Shiffrin, 1968).

Once the sensory memory has processed any new information, the student brain begins to analyze these elements within the working memory (Swellar et al., 1998). Working memory load can be described as the mental effort necessary to accomplish a task or tasks. Historical research on how the brain processes and stores information has shown that working memory can process about seven data elements, plus or minus two, at one time (Miller, 1956). An example in the area of nursing education might be learning how to complete a physical assessment of the cardiac system. Students must apply previous knowledge about the cardiac system that they have learned in their anatomy and physiology (A & P) course and combine it with the newly presented material about the inspection, palpation, percussion, and auscultation needed to learn how to assess the cardiac system. Remember that the student's brain can only process about seven data elements at one time. Clearly there are more than seven data elements to process in the provided example. We are also assuming that students are easily and readily recalling information learned within their cardiac A & P, pathophysiology, and medical terminology courses. The number of elements working memory can process will decrease by about half that if the student is required to analyze, connect, or critically think about the elements rather than just retain them (Cowin, 2001). Using the cardiac assessment example, the student may be asked to connect and critically think about too many things at one time for real learning to occur. Understanding the concept of brain architecture, we as educators can begin to appreciate that "working memory is a paradoxical resource, because it's both the bottleneck and the engine of learning" (Clark & Lyons, 2008, p. 86).

Here is the good news: unlike short-term memory, long-term memory is unlimited in its capacity (Vogel-Walcutt, Gebrim, Bowers, Carper, & Nicholson, 2011). According to CLT theorists, construction of schema can help students to store data into their long-term memories. *Schemas* are models or hypothetical structures that can assist a student in organizing knowledge about the world in which they live (Errey, Ginns, & Pitts, 2006). *Schema construction* promotes storage of information into the long-term memory and can help students not only learn, but also retain what they are taught.

Let's look at an example of a schema. When I teach about cardiac examination, I have the students envision the plumbing of the house. Sometimes I even have them draw on a piece of paper to the best of their ability, the plumbing of a house on a blank sheet of paper. Somewhere within the center of the house, they draw a heart from which all this plumbing originates. When we begin to discuss congestive heart failure, we look at where the "plumbing" is backing up in the "house." When students see how the cardiac system is the same as something they are already familiar with, they can scaffold that information onto preexisting knowledge. This is schema formation. When the student is able to connect something from their long-term memory with newly acquired information, they can store the new information in their brains more easily, and learning and retention of that information occurs at a more rapid pace. This provides just one example of how "chunking" information into a schema can assist with understanding, learning, and retention of any new material. Many times the student will not have a schema on which to scaffold newly acquired knowledge. In this case, a new schema must be developed within the working memory. It makes sense that this will require an increase in mental effort or cognitive load. Within CLT this mental effort is referred to as the germane cognitive load (Swellar et al., 1998).

If we think about these concepts of CLT as we are designing how we will teach, we have to understand that working memory load is affected by two main factors. The first is how complex the material to be learned is (intrinsic cognitive load) and the second is the manner in which we as the instructor teach that material (extraneous cognitive load) (Swellar et al., 1998). These cognitive load principles must be added together to measure the student's cognitive load for learning the material. For example, if the intrinsic nature of the material is low, like memorizing five medical technology terms, extraneous cognitive load can be high without having much effect on student learning. To put it another way, if there isn't much to learn in the first place, or what needs to be learned is simple, we can be really ineffective at teaching the material, and the students will still be able to learn. However, if the student is asked to group these five medical terms together to describe how a disease process occurs and what nursing interventions they should apply, the intrinsic load of the material is increased. If we are not very effective at teaching this kind of complex material to our students (extraneous load), the additive effect of high intrinsic (content) and high extraneous load (teaching) may be too much for student learning to occur.

Unfortunately, the intrinsic cognitive load can't be changed, because it is a result of the type of material being delivered. I would consider most if not all of the material we teach nursing students to have a high or fairly high level of intrinsic load. Here is the good news! Nurse educators have the power to lower extraneous cognitive load for our students and decrease the overall effort it takes for learning to occur. If we engage the students using innovative instructional design, students have the potential to learn complex concepts more easily and be able to retain those concepts for further recall in subsequent nursing coursework much more easily. Thinking about the application of CLT, Benner's Novice to Expert, and Bloom's taxonomy in light of the prospects of the flipped classroom model, we as educators can greatly affect the way in which our students learn within our classrooms. I think that is very exciting news for the nursing education flipped classroom! (The concepts of cognitive load theory described here are only a small part of the overall theory. For more in-depth information, the reader is encouraged to access van Merrienboer and Swellar, [2010].)

So what are Benner and colleagues' ideas for a new vision for nursing education? Well, these authors, also educators themselves, understand that pressure to address the packed nursing curricula we discussed earlier. They believe that this pressure has almost forced nurse educators into "widespread reliance on, as one educator called it, 'canned PowerPoint teaching'" (2010, p. 8). They also note that "where the clinical and classroom instruction are not integrated or coordinated, students report a fragmented experience" (p. 12). A fragmentation within their learning environment can lead students to a superficial understanding and can alter their ability to make perceptive clinical judgments in a variety of patient care situations (2010). Consequently, it can also increase the overall cognitive load and negatively affect learning ability. In short, the way we have been educating in the past, not connecting the students' classroom time to real-life clinical knowledge, can stunt their ability to develop critical thinking skills for their future practice. I don't know about you, but this really bothers me as an educator. I can also see Benner and colleagues' point when I look back over my nursing education. I often would learn about a topic in lecture, but not see a patient with that condition, or have to apply my knowledge to any kind of clinical picture until much later in an experiential, clinical learning environment. I remember having to re-learn much of the information needed for care of the patient when the opportunity did arise.

Now I understand that some of the timing just cannot be helped. We can never guarantee that our student will have a patient with myocardial infarction (MI) the same week that we teach on that content. But we could set up our classroom to require each and every student to apply their knowledge about care of an MI patient within the classroom and move them up the Bloom's taxonomy ladder. In this way, we have a real advantage to be able to help students in a virtually created clinical world right there in our classroom. We don't need a high-fidelity simulator for this classroom experience, although we can add that later on. We can be there with the students, walking them through how to apply their knowledge and think about nursing care, at the bachelor's master's or doctoral level, with the instructor there to guide their thinking.

How is this different than any other interactive or group-based learning? Well, it isn't at first glance. But with the flipped classroom, we have the ability to provide some homework prior to class within the video lecture. When the students come to the classroom, they can then apply that lecture material and any of their assigned readings to get into the heart of the matter, the care of the MI patient. As mentioned previously, this is a great way for us to have our lecture and interactive learning, too. I for one was not ready to let go of my lecture and what I still consider to be a big part of my job in *exchange* for active learning in the classroom. I think we would all agree that trying to apply something we don't understand just leads to frustration and a defeated attitude. What we can do is keep that lecture-type teaching that we've come to revere and give it to the students online where they can use it at their own pace. Then when we have time with them in class, we can be more involved in helping them deepen their understanding and move on to application of rote information in a more active and experiential learning process. I think no one can state it better than Bergmann and Sams, "Flipped learning, at its core, is individualized learning" (2014, p. 7). As Benner and colleagues (2010) say, "classroom teachers must step out from behind the screen full of slides and engage students in clinic-like learning experiences that ask them to learn to use knowledge and practice thinking in changing situations, always for the good of the patient" (p. 14). I hope you are intrigued and ready to learn more about how to implement the flipped learning model into your nursing education classroom.

References

American Association of Colleges of Nursing. (2015). *The AACN essentials for bachelorette education.* Retrieved from http://www.aacn.nche.edu/publications/order-form/baccalaureate-essentials

Atkinson, R. C., & Shiffrin, R. M. (1968). Human memory: A proposed system and its control processes. In K. W. Spence & J. T. Spence, *The psychology of learning and motivation: Advances in research and theory* (Vol. 2, pp. 742–775). New York, NY: Academic Press.

Benner, P. (2001). *From novice to expert: Excellence and power in clinical nursing practice.* Hoboken, NJ: Prentice Hall.

Benner, P., Sutphen, M. Leonard, V., & Day, L. (2010). *Education nurses: A call for radical transformation.* Stanford, CA: The Carnegie Foundation for the Advancement of Teaching.

Bergmann, J., & Sams, A. (2012). *Flip your classroom: Reach every student in every class every day.* Eugene, OR: International Society for Technology in Education.

Bergmann, J., & Sams, A. (2014). *Flipped learning: Gateway to student engagement.* Eugene, OR: International Society for Technology in Education.

Bloom, B. S., Engelhart, M. D., Furst, E. J., Hill, W. H., & Krathwohl, D. R. (1956). *Taxonomy of educational objectives: The classification of educational goals.* New York, NY: David McKay Company, Inc.

CBS News, (2013). More students working (a lot) in college. Retrieved from http://www.cbsnews.com/news/more-students-working-a-lot-in-college/

Clark, R. C., & Lyons, C. (2008). *Graphics for learning: Proven guidelines for planning, designing, and evaluating visuals in training materials.* San Francisco, CA: Pfeiffer.

Cowin, N. (2001). The magical number 4 in short-term memory: A reconsideration of mental storage capacity. *Behavioral & Brain Sciences, 24*(1), 87–114.

Errey, C. Ginns, P., & Pitts, C. (2006, April). Cognitive load theory and user interface design: Making software easy to use. Retrieved from http://www.ptg-global.com/PDFArticles/Cognitive%20load%20theory%20and%20user%20interface%20design%20Part%201%20v1.0.pdf

Finkelman, A., & Kenner, C. (2012). *Teaching IOM: Implications of the institute of medicine reports for nursing education* (3rd ed.). Silver Spring, MD: American Nurses Association.

Hamilton, J. (2008). Think you're multitasking? Think again. Retrieved from http://www.npr.org/templates/story/story.php?storyId=95256794

Institute of Medicine. (2011). *IOM future of nursing report.* Retrieved from http://www.nursingworld.org/MainMenuCategories/ThePracticeofProfessionalNursing/workforce/IOM-Future-of-Nursing-Report-1

Miller, G. A. (1956). The magical number seven, plus or minus two. *Psychological Review, 63,* 50–62.

Northern Virginia Community College. (2015). *What is a hybrid course?* Retrieved from http://www.nvcc.edu/academics/hybrid/student/definition/

Oregon State University. (2015). *Center for teaching and learning: OSU hybrid FAQ's.* Retrieved from http://oregonstate.edu/ctl/osu-hybrid-faqs

Palfrey, J., & Gasser, U. (2008). *Born digital: Understanding the first generation of digital natives.* New York, NY: Basic Books.

Prensky, M. (2010). *Teaching digital natives: Partnering for real learning.* Thousand Oaks, CA: Corwin SAGE.

Statistic Brain Research Institute. (2015). *Attention span statistics.* Retrieved from http://www.statisticbrain.com/attention-span-statistics/

Swellar, J., Ayres, P., & Kalyuga, S. (2011). *Cognitive load theory.* New York: Springer.

Swellar, J., van Merrienboer, J., & Paas, F. (1998). Cognitive architecture and instructional design. *Educational Psychology Review, 10*(3), 251–296.

The Flipped Learning Network. (2014). *What is flipped learning?* Retrieved from http://www.flippedlearning.org/cms/lib07/VA01923112/Centricity/Domain/46/FLIP_handout_FNL_Web.pdf

The George Washington University. (2015). *University teaching and learning center: Hybrid courses.* Retrieved from https://tlc.provost.gwu.edu/hybrid-courses

University of Georgia. (2015). *Sleep rocks, get more of it!* Retrieved from https://www.uhs.uga.edu/sleep/

van Merrienboer, J., & Swellar, J. (2010). Cognitive load theory in health professional education: Design principles and strategies. *Medical Education, 44,* 85–93.

Vogel-Walcutt, J. J., Gebrim, J. B., Bowers, C., Carper, T. M., & Nicholson, D. (2011). Cognitive load theory vs constructivist approaches: Which best leads to efficient, deep learning? *Journal of Computer Assisted Learning, 27,* 133–145.

West LA College. (2015). *What is a hybrid class?* Retrieved from http://info.wlac.edu/hybrid

CHAPTER 2

Evidence-Based Nursing Pedagogy: Show Me the Research!

Introduction

Although the flipped classroom is fairly new to education in general, there is a growing body of research available on its implementation. Unfortunately, not much of the research has been conducted within nursing education, because nursing is one of the more recent professions to dabble with the idea. What is available within the current literature adds valuable information to use of the method within the nursing profession, and will be the first set of studies to be reviewed. The second part of the chapter will review the studies on those professions that are not nursing, but medicine and allied health. Finally, some of the most helpful resources from the Kindergarten through 12 grade level (K-12) realm will be discussed. Because the K-12 educational community has been implementing the method for the longest duration, the suggestions and ideas will be reviewed as contributing to the overall discussion of flipping the classroom. There are also several earlier books from our K-12 pioneers using the method and websites that are full of blogging activity, suggestions, and advice on implementing the flipped classroom. Although much of the activity on these websites is focused on K-12 education, a fair amount is beginning to address higher education as well. Accessing these websites on a regular basis can introduce those interested in the flipped classroom to some new ideas and current technology available.

Table 2-1 Levels of Scientific Evidence

Level	Description of Studies
Level I:	Evidence from a systematic review of all relevant randomized controlled trials (RCTs), or evidence-based clinical practice guidelines based on systematic reviews of RCTs
Level II:	Evidence obtained from at least one well-designed RCT
Level III:	Evidence obtained from well-designed controlled trials without randomization, quasi-experimental
Level IV:	Evidence from well-designed case-control and cohort studies
Level V:	Evidence from systematic reviews of descriptive and qualitative studies
Level VI:	Evidence from a single descriptive or qualitative study
Level VII:	Evidence from the opinion of authorities and/or reports of expert committees

Puddy, R. W., & Wilkins, N. (2011). *Understanding evidence part 1: Best available research evidence. A guide to the continuum of evidence of effectiveness*. Atlanta, GA: Centers for Disease Control and Prevention.

Even though educational research is not typically as rigorous as what we are used to seeing in the health sciences literature, there is a call for ranking of each piece of evidence about the flipped classroom using the same levels of scientific evidence for quantitative research questions. Those in need of a refresher on what each level of research entails, please see **Table 2-1**.

Nursing Research and Articles on Flipped Learning

Although the concept of the flipped classroom is relatively new to nursing education, some nurse educators have applied the flipped classroom or a version of it and were able to publish not only their experiences, but also some preliminary research on the method. Each one of the existing nursing education studies will be reviewed individually and presented from highest to lowest in their scientific rigor.

Flipping the Classroom to Improve Student Performance and Satisfaction—Level III

The review of nursing education research begins with Missildine, Fountain, Summers, and Gosselin (2013), who studied the flipped classroom within two BSN adult health courses. The design of their study most aligns with Level III evidence, as they did randomly assigned their students into three separate groups, but did so within a quasi-experimental education environment. The control group, as you would expect, learned by the typical, traditional lecturing method ($n = 130$). A second group was provided the same lecture in class, but was also able to access a recording of the lecture to review at home at their own convenience ($n = 129$). The third group included students who were instructed with the flipped classroom ($n = 186$) as it was defined earlier in the text. The researchers had two main research hypotheses: (1) The flipped classroom method would result in higher course exam averages than those students who received lecture only and lecture augmented with online recordings and (2) the flipped classroom method would result in higher student satisfaction, and lower student satisfaction would be found in those receiving only lecture and lecture augmented with recordings (2013).

The results were very promising, as exam scores were found to be significantly higher for those students in the flipped classroom group ($M = 81.89$, $SD = 5.02$) than students in both the lecture only ($M = 79.00$, $SD = 4.51$, $p < 0.001$) and the lecture augmented with recordings groups ($M = 80.70$, $SD = 4.25$, $p = 0.003$) (Missildine et al., 2013, p. 598). It is worth mentioning that the scores increased as the student groups were given more control over their learning, although this was not touted as one of the findings of the study by the authors themselves. Students in the flipped classroom group also passed the course at significantly higher numbers than students in the other two groups. In fact, it was found that with use of the flipped classroom, an additional 47 students achieved passing grades in the course (2013).

The second hypothesis of the study was not, however, supported. There were 445 students who completed the researcher-developed satisfaction survey, a 75% response rate. (The fact that the survey lacked predetermined validity was listed as a limitation of the study.) Those students who were in the lecture only and augmented lecture groups had significantly higher satisfaction scores than those in the flipped classroom group. Missildine and colleagues did report that students in the flipped classroom group found this form of instruction to require more work of them as students. The researchers discussed the great potential for the flipped classroom within nursing education, but also believed that faculty may need to refine implementation techniques to "gain students' approval of these new approaches" (Missildine et al., 2013, p. 599).

Using the Flipped Classroom in Graduate Nursing Education—Level IV

Critz and Knight (2013) researched use of the flipped classroom within their graduate Family Nurse Practitioner pediatrics course. The authors felt compelled to change their teaching style after finding in their student evaluations that students were feeling disengaged from and uninvolved in the course. These faculty had been using slide presentations consisting of a combination of student presentations for assignments and more expert faculty lectures. In addition, they had sporadic placement of case studies and group discussions throughout the semester. Using two main exams for learning outcome assessment, the authors found that even though students were passing the course, the grades were not at the level the faculty expected from students at the graduate level.

To redesign their classroom, Critz and Knight had their students complete what they described as a set of modules the week prior to coming to the scheduled face-to-face class time. Within the modules were short lectures that the faculty had recorded using screen capture software along with other videos on the content. The students also had their typical readings from the assigned textbook along with several peer-reviewed, evidence-based journal articles on the content. When all of these steps were completed, the students were required to take a post-test on the content that was primarily application, case study–type questions rather than rote memorization. In total, these post-tests were worth 60% of the entire course grade. The remainder of their grades consisted of 2 examinations worth 20%, a student presentation worth 10%, and participation also worth 10%.

When the class time came, students were busy with faculty applying their content knowledge from the week to intensive case studies, group problem-solving exercises, role play, differential diagnoses, and pharmacologic management of selected disease states. Critz and Knight described the intensive case studies as being presented in an unfolding manner so that the students had a chance to ask questions at each stage until the diagnosis was reached. The in-class work was always related to the pre-class assignments. In some weeks, the researchers did go back to a more traditional lecture format and allowed time for student presentations, which were primarily in lecture format as well.

To determine the students' satisfaction with the flipped classroom, Critz and Knight (2013) polled their 20 students using an anonymous 10-item online survey using a 5-point Likert scale with additional space for students to make comments. Although admittedly not a large number of participants, 60% of the students felt the material covered was extremely worthwhile and 40% felt it was very worthwhile. Similar percentages were reported for the students' thoughts about the readings, student-led lectures, and prerecorded lectures provided by the faculty. Some of the reported student comments were a feeling of being overwhelmed with the amount of work required outside of the classroom due to working full time. I have heard similar comments from my students, and as a result, I tend to keep the offload content the least labor intensive as possible.

These authors felt that their experience with flipping the classroom was an overwhelming success. They saw their students take charge of their own learning and be more engaged within the classroom than when they used straight lecture as their teaching method. Similar to others who have flipped the classroom, they reported an ability to correct student errors in thinking in real time in order to better assess student strengths and weaknesses (Critz & Knight, 2013). I could not agree with this more, and believe it to be one of the most helpful aspects of flipping the classroom that can allow faculty to really help students learn the material. When I used primarily lecture as a teaching method, I never felt 100% comfortable that my attempt to "transfer" information about patient care to my students actually resulted in student learning. In my flipped classroom, the students who do not understand cannot "hide" as easily. Instead, I am able to bring them out of the hiding place of confusion and misunderstanding into a place of learning about patient care. In a very real sense, the flipped classroom has provided a way for me to evaluate student understanding in real time. For me, this is one of the biggest advantages to using the flipped classroom in nursing.

The Use of Flipped Classrooms in Higher Education: A Scoping Review—Level V

Two faculty from the University of South Australia teamed up to provide what is described as a scoping review of the use of flipped classrooms in higher education. Jacqueline O'Flaherty from the School of Pharmacy and Craig Phillips from the School of Nursing and Midwifery used a five-stage framework to analyze the current state of the science about flipping the classroom within the realm of higher education. In the review, 28 articles from 5 different countries were found: 23 within the United States, 2 in Australia, and 1 each from the United Kingdom, Taiwan, and Malaysia. I would highly recommend this article for a nice overview of the state of science regarding flipping the classroom. As you might imagine, the article is full of helpful information and tables of summarization of the available literature. In **Table 2-2** you will find a brief summary of their findings.

Table 2-2 Summary of O'Flaherty and Phillips (2015) Scoping Review

Flipped Classroom Topic of Interest	Summary of Findings from Available Research

Technology and strategies used in pre-class activities	• Prerecorded lectures
	  ○ Podcasts
	  ○ Vodcasts (a video podcast)
	  ○ Screencasts
	  ○ Annotated notes
	  ○ Captured videos
	• Assigned readings to be done prior to class
	• Automated tutoring systems
	• Study guides
	• Interactive videos from online repository (such as Kahn Academy)
	• Case-based presentations
	• Simulations

Activities utilized during face-to-face class time	• Case-based presentations
	• Team-based discussions
	• Panel discussions
	• Debates
	• Smart phone apps and tablets
	• Think pair-and-share activities
	• Clicker questions
	  ○ Individual—quizzes or test of knowledge
	  ○ Team-based quizzes
	• Micro-lectures to address gaps in knowledge

Time, cost, and staffing required	• Lead time for faculty described as intense • Funding for lecture capture to develop "library" of videos • Some institutions have support staff to help faculty flip • Technology team support (usually provided by institution) • Some had little lead time due to use of online video resources rather than creating videos on their own
Who is flipping?	• Nursing • Medicine • Pharmacy • Nutrition • STEM—Science, Technology, Engineering, Mathematics • Humanities • Graduate studies—research methods—statistics • Law and economics

(*Continues*)

Table 2-2 Summary of O'Flaherty and Phillips (2015) Scoping Review (Continued)

Flipped Classroom Topic of Interest	Summary of Findings from Available Research
Pedagogical acceptance of flipped classroom	• Clear expectations for students to decrease frustration • Some students critical of fact they had to take responsibility for their own learning outside of scheduled class time • Number of studies suggest students adapted easily to the flipped classroom • Efficient student adaptation with flipped classroom (as time went on) • Suggestion of introducing flipped learning early on in student studies to build an expectation and culture of self-directed learning • Faculty tend to have positive perception of flipped classroom • Both students and faculty tend to be dependent on lecture method because it is familiar, comfortable, instructor centered, and requires little student engagement • Flipped classroom has potential to increase the frequency and intensity of assignments
Evaluation of indirect and direct educational outcomes	• Very few studies with scientific rigor to show definite improvements in higher order thinking and cognition, problem solving, and critical thinking • Many studies reported an increase in student satisfaction with flipped classroom and active learning during class time • Evidence of increase in academic performance in 5 studies, as measured by improved exam results and course grades when compared to control • Evidence to support an increase in student attendance when flipped classroom is used • Qualitative feedback from student course evaluations suggested improved opportunity for teacher contact time, ability to develop communication skills, preferences for working in teams, active student engagement in the classroom—same students negative about flipped classroom due to increase in their time commitment outside of class • Qualitatively speaking: ○ Flipped model enhanced learning experience, students felt empowered, students felt engaged ○ Promotes more independent learners ○ Increased group collaboration—team work ○ Results in students who are better communicators, with better interpersonal and problem-solving skills • Little to no evidence showing any long-term improvement in educational outcomes—most studies focused at course level rather than curricular perspective

Table 2-2 Summary of O'Flaherty and Phillips (2015) Scoping Review (Continued)

Flipped Classroom Topic of Interest	Summary of Findings from Available Research
Remaining gaps in the literature	• Under-utilization of conceptual frameworks that enable a united approach to flipped classroom • Need for stronger evidence in evaluating student learning outcomes over time • Future research should consider other indicators of student engagement and success in the flipped classroom other than test scores and unvalidated satisfaction surveys

Data from O'Flaherty, J., & Phillips, C. (2015). The use of flipped classrooms in higher education: A scoping review. *Internet and Higher Education, 25*, 85–95.

Using Lecture Capture: A Qualitative Student of Nursing Faculty's Experience—Level VI

Although not focused directly on the flipped classroom, a qualitative study from Reed, Bertram, and McLaughlin (2014) present an interesting perspective from nursing faculty about recording videos and making them available to students outside of the classroom. The authors' university had purchased a fully automated lecture capture program, and as a result, the nursing program decided to have all classroom lectures recorded and provided for students after the class was over. The 14 nursing faculty participants had an average age of 55, considered themselves technology proficient, and had taught on average 17 years in nursing programs. Four focus groups were conducted and questions posed about use of the lecture capture software and remaining concerns. Two themes concerning faculty role and identity and two themes concerned with student learning emerged.

The first of the faculty role themes identified by the authors was *Unsettling/Anxious Beginnings*. Faculty reported feeling unsettled and anxious when using the lecture capture software, and didn't feel that they were given a choice to do so. Instead of being something extra for the students, it was more of an expectation of faculty. Faculty felt the training to use the lecture capture and the actual use of the lecture capture was a lot of work for them. They also voiced a concern about being judged by their more technology-savvy students in the classroom, one stating that she did not want to look dumb in front of her students when she didn't know how to use the technology. However, the focus group participants also reported getting used to the new system after the initial big learning curve, one stating that she didn't even notice it anymore.

The second faculty theme was *An Unwelcome Presence*. The new lecture capture was described as unwanted by the faculty in the focus groups. This unwelcome presence was seen as having the potential to interfere with their connections to students within the classroom setting. It was a theme that the faculty felt threatened by the technology in several ways. One participant wondered where their lectures were going. Where was this historical recording of her "going" on the Internet? Would she be laughed at on popular video streaming websites? Activities and conversations that happened in a classroom lecture were seen as having the potential to be taken out of context if in a video format as well. Faculty reported feeling guarded in the classroom and a sense that privacy was breached and possibly security threatened as well. Things that they might have said in a class not recorded they were hesitant to say. The faculty also had concerns that once their lecture had been "captured" on video, what did they need the faculty for (Alexandre & Wright, 2013)? One might argue that in the flipped model, the expert nurse educator is more necessary than ever. Expert faculty are needed in order to come alongside each student in the classroom and explain difficult concepts with direct connections to patient care. Their ability to answer complex questions from students and help correct errors in thinking are keys to the success of the flipped classroom. When done correctly, the flipping classroom cannot be done without expert faculty to guide the students into a deeper learning experience.

The student learning themes included *Student Learning* and *Promise and Potential*. First of all, some of the faculty in this study were concerned that providing their lectures outside of the class time would result in students missing their classes altogether. In fact, several of the faculty participants reported seeing a dropoff in student attendance with recording of lecture and providing it after class was over. Some participants argued that students needed to be in class for discussions, which did not record well on the screen capture. Others, however, were less adamant about students being in class, stating that at some point faculty need to let go of trying to control student attendance in class. The idea of students as consumers, knowing what they are doing as adult learners, was expressed.

In this theme, one participant asked why students would ever come to class if they could just watch the lecture video and pass the test. This idea does make a point that faculty need to be more than a talking head within the classroom during a lecture. Students are highly intelligent and can at times learn despite the instructional design within the classroom. Why would students need to come to class to watch a faculty member read a slide presentation to them that came directly from their assigned readings? Students can complete readings prior to coming to class where that information can be applied. In class, students should be encouraged to deepen their understanding of the readings. Faculty are charged with helping students unpack more complex ideas and applications of readings and make complicated issues more meaningful. The in class time should be used to engage the brain rather than review the readings on a series of presentation slides.

The second of the student learning themes was *Promise and Potential*. Faculty in the focus groups stated that students found great value in having the lecture material recordings and received student feedback thanking them for doing so on their evaluations. Some of the potential benefits of providing lectures after class included the need for an excused absence (to help students catch up), student preparation for testing, and for the ability to review material at an individual pace. Faculty did want to have more information about how students were using the recordings. One of the participants mentioned that having the recorded lectures available to students decreased the amount of time spent on individual tutoring outside of the classroom. Interestingly, these faculty participants were very positive about having some additional class time to work interactively with students.

Flipping the Statistics Classroom in Nursing Education—Level VI

A smaller study by Todd Schwartz (2014) at the University of North Carolina at Chapel Hill focused on implementation of the flipped classroom for a PhD in a nursing statistics course. The math content lends itself well to the flipped format of lecture at home and the faculty there to help students work through difficult mathematical equations and problem sets. Using his 12 doctoral students, he implemented the flipped model for 2 courses each meeting for 3 hours of face time. The courses involved sequential and cumulative learning and mastery of each topic was considered critical prior to moving on to new content (similar to other content in nursing programs in general).

Although only a small sample was used, the findings included student feedback and outcomes. Students did not score the flipped classroom high after the third week, but this changed when asked again at the end of the semester. The author reminds that at first the students may be against the idea of the flipped classroom, but change this opinion over the time they are exposed to the method. Part of their change in heart may be due to the understanding of how much more they understand and learn the content, despite the additional work and requirement for them to be more engaged in learning.

Flipping the Classroom: A Data-Driven Model for Nursing Education—Level VI

McGowan, Balmer, and Chappell (2014) published a short article about their use of the flipped classroom for continuing education for nurses during the ANCC Annual Symposium on Continuing Nursing Education. The project goals were focused on maximizing learning opportunities within a short period of time (1 day), exposing nurse educators to the flipped model of learning by having them be in the role of learner, and expanding the number of contact hours that could be obtained by combining classroom time with prework assignments. The program involved a series of videos that the nurse educators would watch prior to the symposium. These videos were provided in what was called an e-learning environment and were available 1 month prior to the symposium. Reminders were sent each week during the month prior to the symposium as well, in order to encourage participation.

The design of the study used technology that allowed the researchers to build an e-learning environment complete with videos, searchable library related resources, the ability to take notes, set reminders, and ask questions of faculty. The technology also allowed the researchers to keep track of participant activities in the e-learning environment electronically. In the month prior to the symposium, it was found that 102 nurse educators accessed the system and took 178 notes, set 408 reminders, and searched almost 100 resources. Using the activity on the online system, the researchers were able to tailor the live classroom experiences to complement the online pre-work that was completed. During live sessions, the researchers used case studies and audience response systems to apply material learned during the month prior to the conference.

The researchers found that out of the 124 participants that attended the live sessions, 82% had participated in the e-learning environment. Of those who accessed the online learning prior to the live sessions, 74% reported watching more than 10 videos of the 11 part series. By participating in the online learning environment, 76% reported that they felt better prepared to engage with symposium faculty and to be more active learners. Although an exact percentage was not provided, the researchers stated that the majority of participants felt that the flipped classroom model was an effective educational strategy. Some conclusions of the researchers were that it can be expected that although not all will participate in pre-work, 80% would be very possible. In addition, the researchers felt that planning the in-class work to fit the performance on the e-learning provides an ideal learning environment that can be tailored to the individual learners in any given classroom.

Flipping the Classroom With Team-Based Learning in Undergraduate Nursing Education—Level VI

Della Ratta (2015) used a flipped classroom approach with team-based learning as the primary in-class activity for undergraduate nursing students. The study focused more so on the teaching strategy of team-based learning than it did the flipped classroom. The flipped model was not implemented until the second semester of these students' study, and was only introduced briefly. The author looked primarily at course evaluations, which were more positive in the second semester of learning when the flipped model was introduced. This researcher did not use video within the flipped classroom in favor of a narrated PowerPoint. When used, these narrations were reported as highly valued by the students due to their ability to control the pace, go backwards, and repeat as individually necessary. It was also reported that when team-based learning was used with flipped classroom sprinkled in the mix, the students' scores were significantly higher than with traditional methods of teaching (mostly lecture). It is important to remind the reader that the statement about significantly higher scores was not substantiated by any statistics or evidence within the article.

Della Ratta provided some lessons learned when implementing the team-based learning and flipped classroom, starting with the reminder that new teaching/learning strategies take considerable preparation time for the faculty. Creating the narrated PowerPoints was reported as time consuming and challenging. Writing team application activities also took quite a bit of thought and ingenuity. However, once these were in place, they only required minor revisions and/or updating for the future classes.

Narrating a lecture is much more time consuming than creating a video. In addition, students prefer the video format, because they do not have to take the time to manually click through each slide. The other advantage to the screen capture is in the ease of delivery of the video versus the capability to deliver a narrated lecture. If a video using lecture-capture software is supplied to students, they can download and watch it on any device they choose, which is not possible with narrated lectures using the voice-over feature. Many students use mobile devices and find the video files convenient. The ability to watch the videos at any time without having to click through a set of slides and voice-over files is an advantage of the lecture capture video.

Flipping the Classroom for Student Engagement—Level VII

Alexandre and Wright (2013) both from nursing education programs in New York, implemented the flipped classroom as a result of a super storm in their area. Educational institutions were closed and there were power outages and lack of transportation in the area. In the aftermath of the storm, their school was used to shelter more than 800 people who were displaced by the storm. As a result, the nursing instructors began to reach out to their students using Blackboard, providing recorded lectures and pre-class assignments with the goal of applying that material when the courses resumed at the school. Later when they used the flipped classroom purposefully with their RN-BSN students, they found their students to be well prepared for class and very engaged in the in-class presentations and discussions. In this cohort, students were very happy with the flipped classroom and they had a 100% pass rate in the course.

Although this is not a research-based article, Alexandre and Wright (2013) did provide a basic definition of the flipped classroom as well as advice on how other faculty might implement the method. It is their advice to have a clear understanding of the learning objectives, take time to learn what students do not know and respond to those gaps in knowledge, and maintain flexibility in the classroom setting. Another suggestion was that flipping works best with content or topics that can be explained in 15 minutes or less within video content. Their suggestion was to keep the videos the students will watch at home short and to the point. Alexandre and Wright also recommended using existing technology, communicating clearly with the students about how the flipped classroom will be used. This communication should include clear faculty expectations of students both prior to and within the face-to-face classroom settings. The use of group work was another suggestion, stating that it allowed their students to learn from one another, collaborate, partner, and focus on group problem solving.

In addition to the research above are some resources available in the literature that provide advice on how to flip the classroom in nursing and other health professions. McDonald and Smith (2013a, 2013b) have provided professional development to nurses using the flipped model with great success. Their two-part series in *The Journal of Continuing Education in Nursing* provides their discussion of benefits and strategies as well as some guidance on how to develop podcasts and videos. Similarly, Burns (2012) discussed the use of flipped learning and asynchronous online learning for continuing education in *Critical Care Medicine*. Burns states that the barrier of shift work to the traditional type of learning that has been provided for continuing education (CE) to large groups of employees makes flipped learning and online options for CE a real benefit in delivery of important educational offerings.

Research and Articles on Flipped Learning from Other Professions

It's Not About Seat Time: Blending, Flipping, and Efficiency in Active Learning Classrooms—Level III

In the world of chemistry education, Baepler, Walker, and Driessen (2014) wondered if the seat time for their large chemistry course could be reduced with the use of a flipped classroom. These authors both blended and flipped their classroom, measuring post-test comparisons. One section of their chemistry course was split into three different parts that met only once a week instead of three times a week, while a larger portion of the course's learning activities were moved to the online environment. The main idea was to get more concentrated face-to-face time between students and instructors, even if it occurred only once a week. The face-to-face session would be compared to the traditional lecture-based classroom with the instructor lecturing rather than working with students in small groups. The research hoped to prove that seat time within the classroom would not necessarily mean student learning time due to the quality of interactions rather than the quantity of time involved during face-to-face class time.

At the beginning of the study, student demographics and initial testing were all statistically similar. It was found that flipped, hybrid, active-learning classes that decrease student seat time by two thirds can yield student learning outcomes that are at least as good as, and in one study better than, the traditional full-lecture auditorium class. Importantly, it was also found that the move to the new format did not disadvantage students at any particular grade point average level. Student perceptions of their learning experience improved significantly with the flipped, hybrid format as well. These results beg the question of how much more learning could occur if students were offered the chance to interact and learn directly from instructors each class period rather than cutting class time down by a third. The potential is great, and most students would no doubt enjoy the ability to actively engage with faculty and get their questions answered directly when necessary.

The Flipped Classroom: A Course Redesign to Foster Learning and Engagement in a Health Professions School—Level III

McLaughlin et al. (2014) redesigned a first-year pharmacy course into the flipped classroom at the University of North Carolina Eshelman School of Pharmacy. Their students were required to do a self-paced interactive learning module (called an iLAM), assigned readings, and application exercises prior to coming to class. Each face-to-face class time had a similar structure with 15 minutes of clicker questions using an audience response system, a 15-minute pair-and-share time or micro-lecture, 25 minutes of student presentations including discussions, and finally a 20-minute quiz (individual or paired) over the material of the day. Learning evaluation for the course included three exams, several quizzes, points for engagement, student projects, and a cumulative final exam.

Data were collected on voluntary pre- and post-surveys, which 62 of the 150 students completed. Correlations were also used to show connections between student engagement and their final examination scores. The majority of students reported completing the at-home materials, but correlations between online engagement measures and final exam performance were weak ($r = -0.04$ to $r = 0.20$). There was a higher correlation between the number of online extra credit points that were completed and the final course grade ($r = 0.34$). Students in the flipped classroom were statistically more likely to agree that active student engagement was consistently encouraged ($p = < .001$) and participation was necessary to be successful ($p = < .001$). Attendance was also statistically significantly higher in the flipped classroom ($p = .03$). Students in the flipped classroom also had significantly higher final grades than those in the traditional classroom ($p = < .001$). These researchers also found that students who stated they preferred lecture to active learning prior to the class changed their minds after being a part of the flipped classroom.

The authors also provided some insight from their experiences and feedback of their students about ways to enhance student learning. Believe it or not, they reported no longer considering the textbook as required reading because students found it to be redundant and outdated. They also replaced student presentations with 30-minute active learning exercises and added instructor-administered and graded 20-minute quizzes online outside of class time to insure preparation for class. Student grading of each other's work was added and an online portal of pharmacy information called the "Pharmacopedia" was developed to provide expanding concepts, new technologies, current clinical trials with medications, new drug products, and weblinks.

The Experience of Three Flipped Classrooms in an Urban University: An Exploration of Design Principles—Level IV

Kyu Kim, Mi Kim, Khera, and Getman (2014) from the University of Southern California used a mixed-methods approach to evaluate the flipped classroom within the three different professions of engineering, sociology, and humanities. The three instructors had specialty training and mentors to help them with the development and implementation of the flipped classroom, and had 115 students enrolled in their three courses. Out of these 115 students, 41 students provided responses (36%) to surveys. The researchers also used instructor reflections, interviews, and other documents such as course syllabi. Overall, the researchers reported that their student participants perceived the flipped classroom activities as more student oriented than their traditional classes. Combined data from the three courses were used to develop a design framework for flipped learning. Nine design principles emerged from the data and are provided for review in **Table 2-3**.

Table 2-3 Kyu Kim, Mi Kim, Khera, and Getman's Design Principles for the Flipped Classroom

Design Principles	Description
Provide opportunity for students to gain first exposure prior to class	• Students able to prepare for class ahead of time • Students can learn at their own pace
Provide an incentive for students to prepare for class	• Use low-stakes grading to insure students are prepared • Require students to submit questions/comments on YouTube and give points for doing so
Provide a mechanism to assess student understanding	• Low-stakes quizzes (3–5 questions on learning management system) • Formative assessments
Provide clear connections between in-class and out-of-class activities	• Make sure homework and in-class work focus on same or similar content
Provide clearly defined and well-structured guidance	• Be clear about flipped classroom expectations • Scaffold learning • Give students clear instructions and structure

(Continues)

Table 2-3 Kyu Kim, Mi Kim, Khera, and Getman's Design Principles for the Flipped Classroom (Continued)

Design Principles	Description
Provide enough time for students to carry out the assignments	• Provide adequate time for students to complete in-class activities and online activities • Help students learn self-regulation in their learning
Provide facilitation for building a learning community	• Create learning communities that connect students and help them to collaborate • Group dynamics are difficult and can hinder group work in class and out of class—provide excellent guidelines for groups
Provide prompt/adaptive feedback on individual or group works	• Students desire prompt and specific feedback
Provide technologies familiar and easy to access	• Spend more time on how to integrate technology with pedagogy rather than use of the technology itself

Data from Kyu Kim, M., Mi Kim, S., Khera, O., & Getman, J. (2014). The experience of three flipped classrooms in an urban university: An exploration of design principles. *Internet and Higher Education, 22*, 37–50.

Although many of these authors' design principles seem to be obvious, it is important to listen to the researchers' suggestions in order to avoid making some simple mistakes. These ideas can help faculty to structure their planning for the flipped classroom, and help them to develop a framework of ideas. It is interesting that most of these authors' suggestions focus on providing a clear and straightforward set of expectations for the students, communicating with them clearly about their learning, and using the flipped classroom as a pedagogy that integrates technology rather than being technology centered. It would be safe to argue that with most major changes in process, a clear set of expectations about the new process is a must. This article provides some valuable information about process change, but is not terribly helpful when it comes to implementation of the flipped classroom in real time.

Student Perceptions Toward Flipped Learning: New Methods to Increase Interaction and Active Learning in Economics—Level VI

Noticing the lack of higher education research on the flipped method, Roach (2014) designed a study to measure student perceptions about his economics flipped classroom. Overall, he found on response to surveys, his students were positive about the flipped classroom. The students thought the flipped classroom helped them learn more effectively and that the class was much more interactive than other courses they had taken. Roach also proposed that the use of media (videos to deliver content) may be more efficient and less timely than having students read a standard textbook or listen to a live lecture. Allowing students to prepare for class with rote memorization and basic understanding prior to coming to class allowed Roach more time for interactive learning in the classroom and resulted in deeper learning in a shorter period of time. As have many other researchers, Roach has called for more research on the flipped classroom that spans disciplines and includes quantifiable evidence of its potential to increase student learning.

Enhancing Student Engagement Using the Flipped Classroom—Level VI

A group of nutrition educators have used the flipped classroom and published on how they implemented the model and their students' perception of the method. Gilboy, Heinerichs, and Pazzaglia (2015) from West Chester University of Pennsylvania used a five-item Likert scale plus two open-ended questions on an anonymous survey online to assess student perceptions of the flipped classroom learning environment. In their sample, 72% ($n = 142$) of students responded voluntarily. Out of these participants, 76% preferred the video lecture over the face-to-face lecture, and 64% indicated their preference to participate in-class activities rather than listen to faculty lecture. About the same number of students (62%) felt that they learned material more effectively by viewing the online recorded lectures than when they were in class during a lecture. Some faculty may fear that their students have the potential to feel less connected to them if the flipped classroom is used. These researchers found that 70% of their student respondents felt connected to their faculty when the flipped classroom was used.

The researchers also found that students liked the ability to learn at their own pace and the ability to apply what they were learning with the teachers there to guide them. Curiously, these student participants had some of the same concerns as faculty about some of their peers not being prepared to engage fully in the face-to-face class time activities. With or without using the flipped classroom, insuring active participation by each and every student when using group work is a challenge. The authors provided some solutions to this problem, including an online discussion board prior to class to alert faculty to students who are not doing their part prior to class. They also suggested the faculty do a quick quality check with each group of students at the start of class and then move around to help from group to group as needed.

Also included in this article is a section about lessons learned. The authors discussed their experience with the flipped classroom as rewarding, but warn that the upfront time to make the lectures and develop learning activities requires extensive planning and time. Also suggested is an attempt to gain buy in from the students, use of instructional designers if available, and keeping video-recorded lectures to 15 minutes or less. In addition, they suggest that faculty use course-level analytics available in an online learning system to provide faculty knowledge of accountability and student engagement out of the classroom. They also suggested the use of video resources other than those made by faculty if possible, such as TED talks or Khan Academy videos. Here is where our opinions differ, because I have heard from my flipping colleagues as well as from my students that they much prefer their faculty delivering the video lecture themselves. Although we think that our less-professional video may be less desirable, our students seem to prefer the lectures that we provide and anecdotally prefer our videos.

The Use of Flipped Classroom to Enhance Engagement and Promote Active Learning—Level VI

A study done in Malaysia with instruction technology students attempted to measure various levels of engagement in the flipped classroom with instructional technology students (Jamaludin & Osman, 2014). A study used a small sample of 24 students. The take-home point from this study was that the flipped classroom may help students self-regulate their learning behaviors. This notion makes sense because the students with flipped learning are more able to learn at their own pace and be able to self-regulate rather than be moved methodically along with their cohort. Most educators would agree that in any given cohort or class of students, there exist several different levels of learners. In addition to the levels of learners, there are individual personality traits that affect how a student tends to absorb material. I think back to my own experience with lecturing in the classroom. I talked and delivered information at one pace, but my students could be listening, absorbing the lecture, and learning at a much different pace. When students have the ability to slow down or pause a lecture within the video, they automatically self-regulate their learning.

The Flipped Classroom Paradigm for Teaching Palliative Care Skills—Level VII

Periyakoil and Basaviah (2013) have used the flipped classroom model to teach palliative care skills to medical students at the Stanford University School of Medicine. The lack of experts to mentor medical students about how to deliver expert palliative care coupled with a need for more time in the classroom for discussion and clarification were listed as reasons for using the flipped classroom. The instructors had the students do what they called pre-work in the third quarter of their program including an online video module on theory of and evidence related to discussing bad news with patients and families. They also watched video vignettes of suboptimal examples. During face-to-face time, the students split into small groups and viewed a professionally filmed 5-minute vignette together, then brainstormed on how the interaction could have been improved. After a bit of role play and feedback from their peers, the students watched a professional, more optimal, version of how to discuss bad news with patients.

Although no data was collected during this use of the flipped classroom, the authors provided an example of how medical educators are attempting the flipped model of learning. Much of what has been provided in this case example of the flipped classroom involves working to provide front material and using that within the face-to-face time with students to engage them and make them use and apply what they have learned.

The Changing Landscape of Anesthesia Education: Is a Flipped Classroom the Answer?—Level VII

Kurup and Hersey (2013) reported on their use of the flipped classroom to deliver educational material in anesthesia education. Recognizing the ever-growing time constraints on resident education, the authors discussed the flipped classroom as a way to increase attendance in their class, supplement intraoperative teaching (experiential learning), and limit lecture time in the classroom. They found with their use of the flipped classroom that online learning worked best when combined with face-to-face learning, but did not describe this as a hybrid class. Their students liked the additional time with their faculty in the classroom setting aside from lecture. It was one of their suggestions to use lower order cognitive skills with the online, pre-class learning and step up those cognitive skills when the faculty were there to assist the students. This advice is similar to this book's suggestion and several other resources about flipped learning.

Additional Resources Focused on Flipped Learning

A chapter reviewing the resources available for the flipped classroom would be remiss without the mention of Jonathan Bergmann and Aaron Sams (2012, 2014), the pioneers of flipped learning on the K-12 landscape. These innovative educators have published two books on flipping the classroom and are active in a number of blogs, on YouTube and Twitter. The first of their books was the most helpful to me in my flipping adventures: *Flip Your Classroom: Reach Every Student in Every Class Every Day* (2012). They have since published another book about their new ideas regarding flipped learning: *Flipped Learning: Gateway to Student Engagement* (2014).

Table 2-4 Web-Based Resources on the Flipped Classroom

Website	URL
Flipped Learning Network	http://flippedlearning.org
Edutopia	http://www.edutopia.org
Teacher tube	http://www.teachertube.com
Educational Technology and Mobile Learning	http://www.educatorstechnology.com
Flipped Classroom Workshop	http://www.flippedclassroomworkshop.com
Flipped Institute	http://flippedinstitute.org

Another text that quickly followed Bergmann and Sams first edition was one by Jason Bretzmann (2013) titled: *Flipping 2.0: Practical Strategies for Flipping Your Class.* The text provides a brief introduction by Bretzmann himself, then moves on to chapters by additional K-12 educators who provide examples of their flipped classrooms. It is a wonderful example of flipping for the K-12 classroom, and can provide some ideas to nursing educators about how to engage students in the classroom. There is one chapter focused on technology for students that is very helpful, and worth the read.

In addition to these pioneering texts, more resources have become available. **Table 2-4** lists several valuable Internet resources regarding the flipped classroom. Although some of these are not focused solely on higher education, they are helpful in terms of classroom management and use of technology.

Conclusion

Although we can learn quite a bit from reviewing the resources listed in this chapter, it leaves us with the notion that "to learn we must do." The research about use of the flipped classroom is certain to boom over the next decade. Nursing educators can be a part of the quantitative and qualitative state of educational science if we dare to engage in the scholarship of teaching and learning when implementing the flipped classroom.

References

Alexandre, M. S., & Wright, R. R. (2013). Flipping the classroom for student engagement. *International Journal of Nursing Care, 1*(2), 100–103.

Baepler, P., Walker, J. D., & Driessen, M. (2014). It's not about seat time: Blending, flipping and efficiency in active learning classrooms. *Computers and Education, 78,* 227–236.

Bergmann, J., & Sams, A. (2012). *Flip your classroom: Reach every student in every class every day.* Eugene, OR: International Society for Technology in Education.

Bergmann, J., & Sams, A. (2014). *Flipping learning: Gateway to student engagement.* Eugene, OR: International Society for Technology in Education.

Bretzmann, J. (2013). *Flipping 2.0: Practical strategies for flipping your class.* New Berlin, WI: The Bretzmann Group.

Burns, J. (2012). Critical care in the age of the duty hour regulations: Circadian scheduling, standardized handoffs, and the flipped classroom? *Critical Care Medicine, 40*(12), 3305–3306.

Critz, C. M., & Knight, D. (2013). Using the flipped classroom in graduate nursing education. *Nurse Educator, 38*(5), 210–213.

Della Ratta, C. B. (2015). Flipping the classroom with team-based learning in undergraduate nursing education. *Nurse Educator, 40*(2), 71–74.

Gilboy, M. B., Heinrerichs, S., & Pazzaglia, G. (2015). Enhancing student engagement using the flipped classroom. *Journal of Nutrition Education and Behavior, 47*(1), 109–114.

Jamaludin, R., & Osman, S. A. (2014). The use of a flipped classroom to enhance engagement and promote active learning. *Journal of Education and Practice, 5*(2), 124–131.

Kurup, V., & Hersey, D. (2013). The changing landscape of anesthesia education: Is flipped classroom the answer? *Current Opinion in Anesthesiology, 26,* 726–731.

Kyu Kim, M., Mi Kim, S., Khera, O., & Getman, J. (2014). The experience of three flipped classrooms in an urban university: An exploration of design principles. *Internet and Higher Education, 22,* 37–50.

McDonald, K., & Smith, C. M. (2013a). The flipped classroom for professional development: Part I. Benefits and strategies. *The Journal of Continuing Education in Nursing, 44*(10), 437–438.

McDonald, K., & Smith, C. M. (2013b). The flipped classroom for professional development: Part II. Making podcasts and videos. *The Journal of Continuing Education in Nursing, 44*(10), 486–487.

McGowan, B. S., Balmer, J. T., & Chappell, K. (2014). Flipping the classroom: A data-driven model for nursing education. *The Journal of Continuing Education in Nursing, 45*(11), 477–478.

McLaughlin, J. E., Roth, M. T., Glatt, D. M., Gharkholonarehe, N., Davidson, C. A., Griffin, L. M., Esserman, D. A., & Mumper, R. J. (2014). The flipped classroom: A course redesign to foster learning and engagement in a health professions school. *Academic Medicine, 89*(2), 1–8.

Missildine K., Fountain R., Summers, L., & Gosselin K. (2013). Flipping the classroom to improve student performance and satisfaction. *Journal of Nursing Education; 52*(10), 597–599.

O'Flaherty, J., & Phillips, C. (2015). The use of flipped classrooms in higher education: A scoping review. *Internet and Higher Education, 25*, 85–95.

Periyakoil, V. S., & Basaviah, P. (2013). The flipped classroom paradigm for teaching palliative care skills. *Virtual Mentor, 15*(12), 1034–1037.

Puddy, R. W., & Wilkins, N. (2011). *Understanding evidence part 1: Best available research evidence. A guide to the continuum of evidence of effectiveness*. Atlanta, GA: Centers for Disease Control and Prevention.

Reed, P. E., Bertram, J. E., & McLaughlin, D. E. (2014). Using lecture capture: A qualitative study of nursing faculty's experience. *Nurse Education Today, 34*, 598–602.

Roach, T. (2014). Student perceptions toward flipped learning: New methods to increase interaction and active learning in economics. *International Review of Economics Education, 17*, 74–84.

Schwartz, T. A. (2014). Flipping the statistics classroom in nursing education. *Journal of Nursing Education, 53*(4), 199–206.

CHAPTER 3

The Intentional Instruction Model

Origination of the Intentional Instruction Model

Conceptual models and/or frameworks have been used by clinicians and educators to make sense of concepts and provide a template for approaching any particular context. More specifically, a conceptual model has been defined as a type of diagram showing relationships between a set of factors that are believed to lead to a target condition or outcome (Conceptual model, 2015). It became clear during the first attempts to implement the flipped classroom in nursing courses that premeditated, careful organization was essential to success. Having a guideline or some sort of template to follow when attempting to flip the classroom would have been extremely helpful. After an exhausting search of the current literature on flipping the classroom, anecdotal experiences and elementary educational tips were all that were found. There was little to guide novice flipping nursing faculty in the pedagogy.

Most might agree that without any sort of template to work from, initial attempts at flipping the classroom are unorganized at best. Although great enthusiasm and some basic ideas were readily available, none had been tested or tried. Some experiences with flipped classes seemed to be more successful than others. Some would flow very easily with happy students and great learning outcomes during evaluation. But other times the activity floundered, due to lack of experience, preparation, and forethought. There was also a sense of struggling with how to assess or measure the outcomes of the flipped classroom in general. Even though this new teaching and learning strategy was being implemented, there was not a tandem cange in different student assessments of learning. In addition to student learning outcomes, instructor success or need for improvement with use of the method itself were not really being paid attention to. Other than some anecdotal feedback from individual students, there was little to inform one of success or failure as a flipping instructor. All of these issues culminated in the idea that others wanting to implement the flipped classroom within nursing education may be facing similar kinds of challenges.

After being introduced to the flipped classroom during a faculty development provided on the University of Northern Colorado (UNC) campus by the Center for Education Teaching and Learning (CETL), the adventure with flipping began. Our university holds a strong focus on excellent teaching, and has several faculty development opportunities throughout the year to help faculty learn about new and exciting teaching and learning strategies. Dr. Jerry Overmyer, who at the time was a doctoral student in mathematics, presented a session to the campus faculty about the flipped classroom in the fall of 2012. It didn't take much convincing toward a quick decision that this was a teaching and learning method taylor made for nursing education.

Teaching primarily in the Family Nurse Practitioner (FNP) program, I and some of my colleagues had struggled with a lack of time to adequately teach all the content in the curriculum. The faculty teaching this group of students wanted and planned to engage students in interactive learning activities, but rarely had the time to do so after the planned lecture was over. The FNP course objectives were all high-ordered learning, so even when lecture was used, it seemed to leave students needing more application of the material and less listening about the material. Of course, this meant active learning activities to allow the students to engage with the content and practice applying their ideas. It was not unusual to use case-based learning, but the time to do so was always limited. Increasing credit hours within the FNP curriculum was not an option. Faculty were left with a need to engage students within higher ordered learning objectives, couple with a lack of time to do so and use lecture as the main teaching approach.

After attending Dr. Overmyer's session and doing some reading about flipped learning, it was clear that the flipped classroom had primarily been applied to K-12 classrooms. I talked with my teaching colleague Kat Johnson and introduced her to the idea of flipping our FNP course the next semester focused on pediatric and obstetric care. She thought the idea had potential, and we agreed to flip the entire course. We met with the group of students we would be teaching and told them about the flipped classroom. We notified the students that we would be using the flipped classroom in their next FNP course in the spring. In hindsight, we did not prepare them well enough, which led to the chapters in this book about preparation of both faculty and students for the flipped classroom. We did not take into account what we know to be true about change theory. Instead, we assumed the students would be happy to be engaged in this new adventure with us. We quickly were reminded that change is difficult and many times met with resistance, particularly when change is dictated rather than championed.

Using our experiences during that first flipping semester, Kat and I developed and presented a faculty development session for our campus about our experiences using the flipped classroom in the Fall of 2013. It was very well attended, and a topic of interest to many faculty across a variety of different disciplines. That presentation led to another similar podium presentation at the National Organization of Nurse Practitioner Faculties (NONPF) in the Spring of 2014. There we met a few other nursing instructors who were implementing the flipped classroom, and found that we were all engaging in similar techniques with slight differences. The number of faculty who approached us after our session to ask questions and get advice on their development ideas made us realize that several other nursing faculty were recognizing the potential of this method within nursing education.

Because of my experience of being the pioneer of the flipped classroom in nursing in my geographic area, I was invited to be a pre-conference speaker for the Rocky Mountain Nurse Educators Conference in Breckenridge, Colorado the summer of 2014. The conference planners wanted a "how to" session, and scheduled an intensive 4-hour preconference with a focus on how to implement the flipped classroom in nursing education. Kat agreed to help me with the presession, because she had also implemented the flipped classroom within her undergraduate pediatrics course with great success. My experience with flipping included courses in the FNP program, graduate research courses, and undergraduate and graduate physical assessment courses.

While preparing for the conference, I reviewed all of the available literature for flipping within the health professions and beyond that was available at that time. During this search of literature, I realized that the literature provided quite a bit of advice and anecdotal experiences of flipping the classroom, but very little research. In addition, there was not a clear conceptual framework or template to work from for those who wanted to engage in the flipped classroom. With all of the wonderful, and sometimes painful, lessons learned about flipping, it was apparent that a conceptual framework would be essential to helping other nursing faculty flip their classrooms successfully. See **Figure 3-1**.

When developing the first rendition of the conceptual framework, the focus was on creating something straightforward and easy to apply to the nurse educator's setting. Similar to the concept of discharge planning, the ideas started with the end in mind, creating each part of the framework with the focus on excellent student outcomes and the use of intentional instruction. The model was designed so

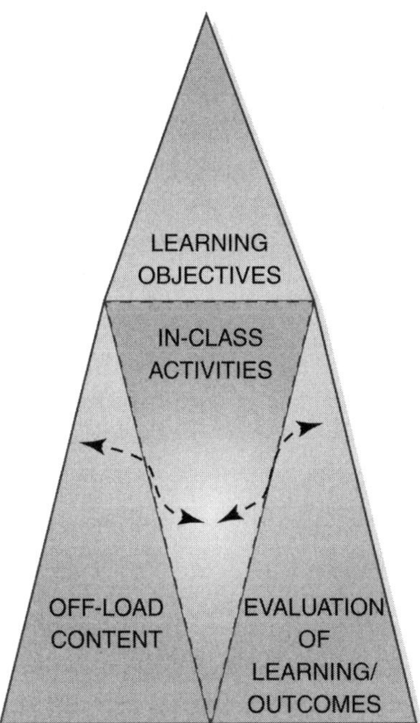

Figure 3-1 Intentional Instruction Model for flipping the classroom.

that program and course objectives sat at the top of the framework, because instructional design should always flow from the predetermined obejctives for learning. Every part of the model was developed with the idea that instruction of students be intentional within the flipped classroom. The model takes the educator out of a "star role" as a lecturer attempting to transfer information to student learners. Instead, the model shows a teaching and learning atmosphere where the faculty *talk with their students* and engage with them intentionally to *teach* the content matter in a different, student-centered manner. As Eric Mazur of Harvard University has depicted, higher education faculty tend to put a great deal of emphasis on transfer of information to student groups (Berret, 2015). As sources of information have become more bountiful and technology more available, the lecture model of teaching where the focus is primarily on transfer of information from faculty to student is becoming a less relevant form of instruction in the modern higher education classroom. As Mazur discussed, transmitting information from faculty member to student during a traditional lecture should no longer be the focus of teaching. Instead, the faculty role in higher education needs to shift to the role of helping students assimilate information (2015). Michael S. Palmer, an associate professor of chemistry at the University of Virginia, has provided the notion that content is no longer going to be the "thing" we focus on as instructors. Instead, our role will be to help each student unpack difficult content for individual student learning to occur (Berrett, 2015). Thinking of all of these aspects of flipped learning, the model was titled, The Intentional Instruction Model for the Flipped Classroom.

The first rendition of the model was focused on personal experience using the flipped classroom and on the current literature available. In order to help others plan to implement the flipped classroom, a conceptual model to help guide each part of the flipping process was developed. It was so serendipitous to read the scoping review by Jacqueline O'Flaherty and Craig Phillips (2015) from the University of South Australia stating that one of the gaps in the literature was a lack of conceptual frameworks for the flipped classroom. Specifically stated:

> *. . . under-utilization of conceptual frameworks that enable a united approach to pre-, face to face and post-learning activities, resulting in a lack of clarity and heavy content focus; an under-developed capacity to blueprint, that is, to translate conceptual frameworks into content-specific plans and a lack of understanding of how to design and support inquiry-based learning and metacognition in a flipped learning curriculum (2015, p. 94).*

The goal of the conceptual model presented in this chapter is to fill the gap identified by O'Flaherty and Phillips. Although the model was developed by a nursing educator with nursing education in mind, the concepts have the potential to be transferrable to other educational foci.

As you can see in Figure 3-1, the original model included the main parts of flipping the classroom: learning objectives, off-load content (what the student would do prior to class), in-class activities, and evaluation. As the model indicates, planning for the flipped classroom begins with the learning objectives, depicted at the top. The learning objectives should guide the rest of the flipped classroom process. In the lower part of the original model are the off-load, in-class, and evaluation parts of the flipped classroom. The model was designed to show how these are all related and can at times overlap. The broken lines between each indicate that they can also fluctuate depending on the learning objectives. For example, one class may have more off-load content, in-class activities, or evaluation of learning one week than the next depending on the topic and course plan.

The original model was helpful toward the goal to teach the flipped classroom planning to fellow nursing instructors at the conference, and resulted in a publication about the flipped classroom process (Hessler, 2015). Continued use of the flipped classroom pedagogy has brought about personal reflection about what actually was implemented in each flipped classroom and course. With more and more research available on the flipped classroom, the model was revised and updated to fit current implementation and state of science.

Revision of the Original Model

Revision of the Intentional Instruction Model took place early in 2015 (**Figure 3-2**). The basic tenets of the model were the same, but a couple of elements were in need of revision after further implementation and exploration of the literature. All of the different facets of the model are those believed to be essential when attempting to flip the nursing classroom. Because each part of the model has its own intricacies, the book has been designed to elaborate on each part of the model within the chapters to follow.

Now before interest is lost with the mention of a theoretical or conceptual model, think of this as a road map or template from which the flipped classroom can be planned for and implemented. Like any good map, it has been designed to help arrive at the destination of a

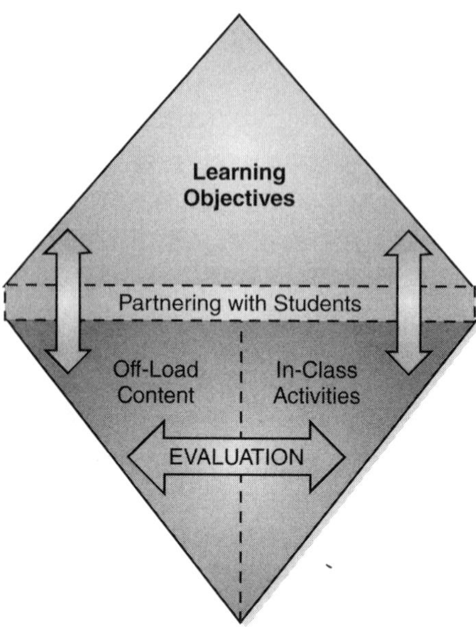

Figure 3-2 Revision of the Intentional Instruction Model for flipped learning.

successful flipped classroom while avoiding the timely detours, painful potholes, and frustrating road blocks along the way. The different concepts and facets of the revised model, how they fit together, and how all parts of the model are fundamental for a success plan to implement the flipped classroom are introduced next.

Learning Objectives

At the top of the model are the ***Learning Objectives*** (**Figure 3-3**) for the material to be using within the flipped classroom. As any educator would probably agree, planning for student learning should flow from the learning objectives for the program, course, or the unit for the day. If the learning objectives do not lend themselves to the flipped learning format, it should not be used. As Bergmann and Sams (2012) have recommended, do not use technology solely for technology's sake. In other words, don't make a video and flip the classroom if it is not content that is conducive to flipping. Lecture is not a dirty word. It is not suggested that faculty never lecture again. On the contrary, many times lecture is

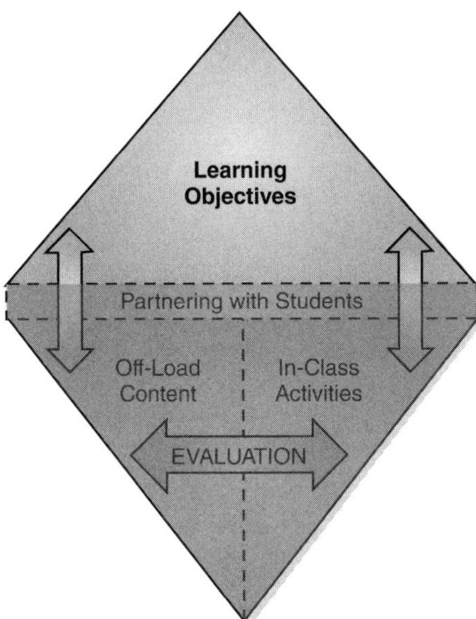

Figure 3-3 Learning objectives.

a necessary component of instructional design, and is still a part of the flipped classroom model. The lecture is simply moved to the individual learning space via videos prior to students coming to the face-to-face class. Even within the flipped classroom, faculty will find themselves at the front of the classroom from time to time to go over a concept that most students struggle with during the in-class activities. Some flipping instructors have called these "micro lectures." Lecturing is certainly not a poor instructional method, but it is suggested that it is one that has been over used in many nursing education settings. The coming chapters will introduce some ways that objectives can be written to reflect the hierarchy within Bloom's taxonomy. Doing so will allow structure for the type of learning students will complete within the off-load and in-class time frames.

Partnering With the Students

Within the first rendition of the model, it was apparent that the students were left out of the planning and implementation of the

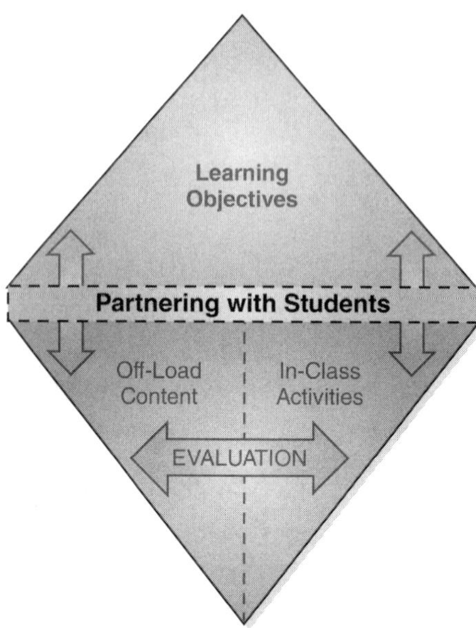

Figure 3-4 Partnering with students.

flipped classroom. Gaining more experience as a flipped classroom educator allowed for more efficiency and success at gaining student acceptance for the teaching/learning method. The result was a need to add students into the model as a central component to successful flipping of the nursing education classroom (**Figure 3-4**). As the literature will show, students in higher education classrooms tend to be more resistant to the idea of the flipped classroom for a variety of reasons. After they are given a chance to experience the flipped classroom and understand how it can help their learning, they can become more accepting of its use. It is not long before faculty realize that they would be wise to partner with their students in the process of implementing the flipped classroom.

In reflection of how my work as an educator and nurse practitioner are similar, I realized that an essential component of my approach to patient care should also be an essential part of the way I educate students. When working with patients and families, it is not good practice to simply dictate the plan of care without asking for input and buy-in. The result is a partnership where practitioner and patient come together to form a plan that works for everyone. When working with patients, I share an analogy for how I can help them be healthy. I tell them that their health is like a ship. The patient is the captain of their health ship. The nurse practitioner is like the navigator for that health ship. It is not the nurse practitioner's job to steer the ship. It is the nurse practitioner's job to give the patient advice on how to steer the ship in the path of good health. If the nurse practitioner sees an iceberg in the health ship path, the nurse practitioner will notify the patient immediately and give advice on how to avoid that iceberg. The nurse practitioner will at no time be driving the patient's health ship—that is the patient's job. The nurse practitioner is not allowed to drive the ship because he or she is not the captain. Only the patient can steer the ship toward health. Therefore, the patient is the "boss" of the ship, and is the only one who can make the ship move or change direction. If the nurse practitioner gives the patient directions as the navigator and the patient chooses not to follow those directions, there is a higher likelihood of having problems with the healthship. Again, the nurse practitioner cannot make the patient steer the ship in the direction he or she is advising. The nurse practitioner wants each patient's ship to be in excellent shape. Remember, only the patient has the power to keep their ship in excellent shape.

Patients tend to understand this analogy, and hopefully it provides a sense of confidence and ability for them to take their health where they want to it to go. Of course, there are always those patients who drive their ship into the fog of smoking or other bad choices, but all the nurse practitioner can do is help them try to get out of that fog. If they don't want out of the fog, the nurse practitioner can't make them get out of the fog. The point is, nurse practitioners cannot dictate or make people do what they want them to do, they can only advise. Once I gave up that desire to control my patients and make them do what I thought was right, it changed the way I looked at patient care. That same sort of thought process and analogy with students in the role as a nurse educator can serve to provide a partnering environment in the classroom.

Nursing students are after all adult learners, and each is the captain of their own learning ship.

Prensky's (2010) work on partnering for real learning addresses the need for faculty to find their niche in teaching the digital native students of the day. In his view, partnering with students involves a new paradigm of thinking about education. He describes partnering within this context: "letting students focus on the part of the learning process that they can do best, and letting teachers focus on the part of the learning process that they can do best" (p. 13). This concept of partnering resonates with me, because it is parallel to the analogy above. He expands this definition to include which things he believes both students and faculty to have primary responsibility for (see **Table 3-1**).

After reviewing the literature and including Prensky's ideas about partnering, it seemed important that partnering with the students within a flipped classroom be an essential part of flipping success. Within my earliest flipped classroom, I had expected my students to be immediately "on board" with my choice to test out the flipped

Table 3-1 Prensky's Teacher and Student Partnering Responsibilities

Students' Primary Responsibility	Teacher's Primary Responsibility
Finding and following their passion	Creating and asking the right questions
Using available technology	Giving students guidance
Researching and finding information	Putting material to be learned into context
Answering questions while sharing their thoughts and opinions	Explaining concepts and material one on one
Practicing (when properly motivated)	Creating rigor in the educational process
Creating presentations in text and multimedia	Ensuring a quality educational process

Developed using Prensky, M. (2010). *Teaching digital natives: Partnering for real learning*. Thousand Oaks, CA: Corwin SAGE.

classroom *on them* rather than working in partnership *with them* to implement the teaching and learning method. Partnering with the students has the potential to help foster buy-in and allow for an easier transition in order to accept a change in their educational experience. Even though the digital native community has been quoted as saying that they do not want to be lectured to, they know little other methods of instruction from their past experiences in the classroom. Therefore, flipping instructors have experienced almost immediate student resistance to the idea of flipping the classroom when it has been dictated to students. Providing a partnering environment where faculty and students decide as a group how the process will unfold presents a much more collegial idea. These students will, after all, be nursing colleagues. Providing some decision making, however small, could go a long way in the acceptance of the flipped classroom for an otherwise resistant group of students. More suggestions on how to partner with the students and share some faculty "educational power" with students can be found later on in the text.

Off-Load Content

The ***Off-Load Content*** portion of the model (**Figure 3-5**) represents any work that students will be assigned to do prior to coming to the face-to-face class. Although many educators using the flipped classroom are using video-recorded lectures, this is not the only way to off-load content. Just as in a traditional lecture course, the instructor is likely to assign students readings to help them meet the learning objectives. Additional off-load content should be carefully planned to reflect not only the learning objectives, but also the amount of time that students will spend preparing for the face-to-face class. There are some faculty who think the flipped classroom will allow them to cover more content than in their traditional lecture format. When asked how this might look, they describe how they can do twice the lecture now that students can watch one or two video lectures at home in addition to the one or two they will deliver within the live classroom. This is not the flipped classroom at all. The flipped classroom is a teaching method focused on helping students gain a

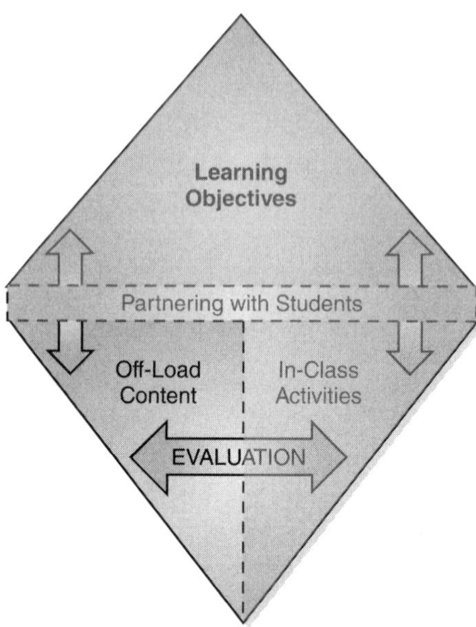

Figure 3-5 Off-load content.

deeper understanding of how to assimilate and apply material they learn prior to coming to class. It is not designed to double the work of the students at home in order to cover more content in the same format, but in a different location. Although this is a very tempting idea, faculty would be wise to avoid using the flipped classroom as a label for doubling student workload. Later on in the text, some solid guidance on how to develop and implement off-load content for ultimate flipped classroom success will be discussed.

In-Class Activities

Perhaps one of the most important parts of the model is the ***In-Class Activities*** (**Figure 3-6**). These activities should be designed to allow the student to work at applying and synthesizing the material assigned in the off-load content. The flipped classroom model can help close the classroom-clinical divide and fragmentation often seen in nursing educational settings described by Benner and colleagues (2010). Therefore, the in-class activities should be chosen carefully and reflect the clinical scenarios and critical thinking that will be

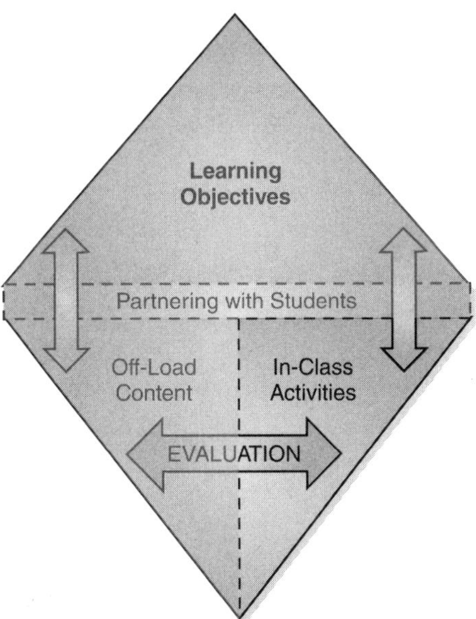

Figure 3-6 In-class activities.

necessary for nursing students to implement while in practice. Careful planning of the in-class activities has the potential to maximize student ability to react in patient care scenarios, understand the hierarchy of patient care, and engage in a clinical setting more readily.

Although there is no research to date to support this concept, it is theorized by Benner's (2001) Novice to Expert theory that if students are able to practice in low-fidelity patient care situations, they will be more prepared to carry out the correct nursing interventions within the actual clinical environment. For this theoretical reason, the in-class activities chosen should closely mimic what is done in practice, and allow faculty to help the students walk through patient care scenarios with an expert nurse at their side. Activities requiring students to engage in group work and team-based learning are helpful. As the research has shown, these types of activities can help students with communication skills. In-future chapters, the text will delve deeper into how to plan for the in class timeframe of the flipped classroom.

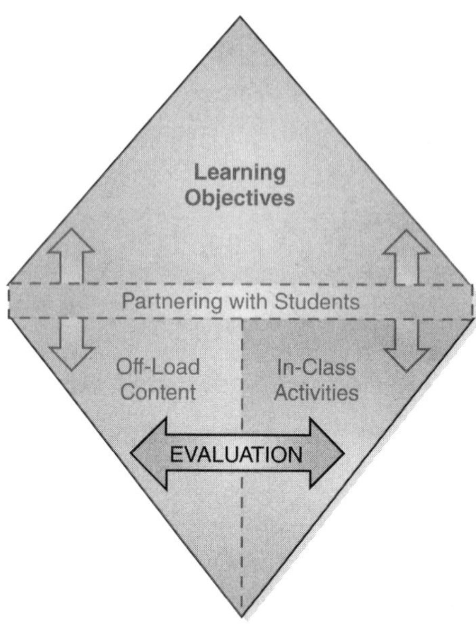

Figure 3-7 Evaluation.

Evaluation

The ***Evaluation*** (**Figure 3-7**) piece of the flipping puzzle in the original model was too isolated to fit what is really needed for successful flipping and learning. Evaluation is not an isolated piece of the flipping experience. On the contrary, the entire process fits within an evaluation plan. There are many different aspects of evaluation to consider when flipping the classroom. After using the flipped classroom more and more, it became clear that evaluation was multifaceted, and needed more consideration within the model to translate into better practice. Evaluation within the Intentional Instruction Model includes evaluation of off-load content, in-class activities, and content learning objective evaluation overall. From a curricular view, evaluation takes a broader scope to include program and curricular outcomes as well. In this respect, it is clear that evaluation should permeate any teaching and learning strategy within a curricular framework. Obviously the evaluation piece must tie back into the predetermined learning objectives. Whether evaluation is used in a formative, on-going manner, or a more summative manner, it requires attention for continuous quality improvement in teaching and learning.

It is through evaluation of teaching that nursing faculty can become more refined, fine-tuned educators. How faculty use self-reflection during and after use of the flipped classroom could be the difference between revising and trying again, and abandoning this form of teaching all together. It is safe to say that many of the teaching techniques attempted are not golden right out of the gate. The focus should be on what was good and bad about the particular implementation at that point in time. Using this information to learn about how to revise and try again is part of eventual success. I certainly felt like quitting the first time I flipped for several reasons. But the potential for better student outcomes was the carrot on the stick that kept me trying. The fact that I really believe that the lecture method is ineffective for many reasons has also been a continual driving force. Even though the evidence about the digital native indicates that they do not want to be lectured to, it is a fact that the majority of nursing students have been taught with lecture most, if not all, of their academic careers. Lecture is what students are used to and what they have grown to expect. We all know that change is difficult, particularly when that change means the student will need to engage with their learning in the classroom rather than taking their comfortable passive role within the lecture seat.

Conclusion

The Intentional Instructional Model for the Flipped Classroom was developed to provide a framework for implementation and evaluation of the flipped classroom. The chapters to follow will expand each of the concepts within the model, including a discussion of the literature to support each concept. The ability to clearly think about each step of the flipped classroom can augment the process and help faculty to be as effectual as possible with the teaching method. Within each of the following chapters, a careful and deliberate planning process will be presented to help you flip your own classroom with success.

References

Benner, P. (2001). *From Novice to expert: Excellence and power in clinical nursing practice.* Menlo Park, CA: Addison-Wesley Pub. Co. Nursing Division.

Benner, P., Stuphen, M. Leonard, V., & Day, L. (2010). *Education nurses: A call for radical transformation.* Stanford, CA: The Carnegie Foundation for the Advancement of Teaching.

Bergmann, J., & Sams, A. (2012). *Flip your classroom: Reach every student in every class every day.* Eugene, OR: International Society for Technology in Education.

Berret, D. (2015). How "flipping" the classroom can improve the traditional lecture. *The Chronicle of Higher Education.* Retrieved from http://chronicle.com/article/How-Flipping-the-Classroom/130857/

Conceptual model. (2015). Dictionary.com. Retrieved from http://dictionary.reference.com/browse/conceptual-model

Hessler, K. (2015). Flipping the classroom in nursing education. *The Journal of the American Academy of Nurse Practitioners.* In press.

O'Flaherty, J., & Phillips, C. (2015). The use of flipped classrooms in higher education: A scoping review. *Internet and Higher Education, 25,* 85–95.

Overmyer, J. (2012, November). *The flipped classroom: Using teacher created online video to increase student engagement.* Greeley, CO: Faculty Development, University of Northern Colorado, Center for Excellence in Teaching and Learning.

Prensky, M. (2010). *Teaching digital natives: Partnering for real learning.* Thousand Oaks, CA: Corwin SAGE.

CHAPTER 4

Faculty Preparation for the Flipped Classroom

Introduction

The decision to try a new and unfamiliar pedagogy can be quite overwhelming. The goal of this chapter is to help faculty expertly prepare for the new teaching and learning strategy of flipping the classroom. Before discussing some ways to prepare for the flipped classroom, the chapter will address the overall attitude of nurse educators about the method. There seems to be an overarching theme of faculty reflected in the available literature that flipping the classroom is too much work, is not proven to be effective, and takes too much time. Anecdotally, faculty have voiced resistance to the idea of the flipped classroom due to the lack of convincing evidence that it is worth that time and effort. One can understand the resistance to change in general, particularly when accompanied by the potential for more work. I find myself wondering then if the resistance of faculty to the flipped classroom has more to do with resistance to change itself rather than resistance to the flipped classroom.

Why the Resistance to the Flipped Classroom?

Any major change in teaching and learning strategy comes with its fair share of preparation and planning. Consequently, it is reasonable to expect some preparation and planning time with implementation of the flipped classroom. It is important to point out that *any change* necessitates a certain amount of preparation and planning. Any time a change is required, there might be a certain amount of natural resistance. Change requires greater amounts of work and energy before, during, and after the change. Maybe this is why some faculty begin to make awful groaning sounds when the words *curriculum* and *revision* are used in the same sentence. The flipped classroom takes a significant amount of time and commitment by the nurse educator, but given a chance, the pedagogy can provide a brand new way to interact more efficiently and effectively with students.

Where does resistance to change originate, exactly? Lisa Quast (2012), an author, career coach, business consultant, and former Fortune 500 executive believes that there are five main reasons people are resistant to change. The first of these reasons is *fear of the unknown*. When change is implemented without warning, those affected by the change are more likely to be resistant. One goal of this text is to provide personal experiences with the flipped classroom coupled with good planning and preparation to decrease nurse educators' fear of the unknown when it comes to flipping the classroom. The following chapter shares some ideas about how to decrease this fear of the unknown among nursing students as well. We can largely avoid student resistance by spending adequate time helping them understand the pedagogy. Students, much like faculty, need to fully understand the flipped classroom process and be assured that the method is worth the discomfort of change prior to buying into the notion. If students and faculty don't have a good understanding of how they will be affected by the change in pedagogy, they are more likely to resist the change due to fear of the unknown.

Mistrust is another reason for resistance to change. According to Quast (2012), if the person making the change is well known and trusted, the change is more likely to be accepted. However, if the person suggesting change does not have an established relationship with those invested in the change, resistance is likely to occur. Faculty can trust in this pedagogy even without stacks of empirical evidence to show that it works. I have witnessed this mistrust and resistance in several faculty members when presenting the method at educational conferences. Faculty want to see solid research that the method is effective, and use the lack of evidence available as a foundation for rejecting the concept of the flipped classroom. There is a common mistrust of anything that hasn't been proven by research in the healthcare arena. The need for evidence prior to implementing healthcare interventions on patients is certainly expected within the current paradigm of evidence-based practice in nursing. The idea of being evidence based is extremely important; however, new pedagogies that have promise must be tried and perfected at some point in the research trajectory. Perhaps attempting to use the method without a stack of empirical evidence to prove its effectiveness is acceptable. As far as I know, compelling research that proves the use of lecture as the main pedagogy is the best way for students to learn is not available either. Therefore, it could be argued that some may be holding onto tradition rather than teaching in an evidence-based manner anyway. There is a perfect opportunity to engage in data collection with any change in pedagogy in order to build the state of science that teaching methods have promise to improve learning within the profession of nursing. As nurse scientists, we should be engaged in the scholarship of teaching and learning in order to build the evidence base regarding best practices for teaching and learning in nursing education.

If those expected to change experience *a loss of control*, resistance to change is more likely (Quast, 2012). Many faculty might admit that they like to lecture because they have better control of their classroom. Some may not like group work and interactive learning because it produces a bit of chaos within the normally quiet and controlled classroom when lecture is the main pedagogy. Those who have grown accustomed to a certain amount of order and control that lecture affords are more likely to resist the interactivity that the flipped classroom requires.

When reflecting on my own experiences in nursing education as both student and instructor, the main focus was on the faculty. The main pedagogy used was lecture when I was a student, and I found myself more comfortable with this type of classroom atmosphere. As a new nurse educator, I remember spending hours ahead of the live class time preparing for the lecture with perfected slides, and applicable examples for the students. A great deal of time was spent in the attempt to make the lecture slides as captivating as possible. I did attempt some interactive activities during classes, but always felt that they could only be done as "extra" on top of the lecture. The lecture was the star of the show and just had to be finished before any time could be spent on interactive learning activities. After some expanded education on how the human brain actually learns, I began to realize that this was not the best thing for the students in my classroom. Although I felt comfortable with my long-held tradition of lecture, it was at the cost of effective teaching and learning.

It might be difficult for some nursing faculty to let go of the nice, controlled order to the classroom that lecture allows. The nursing faculty have the most power in this type of environment. It is what some have become more comfortable with and what the students feel comfortable with as well. So why do nurse educators continue

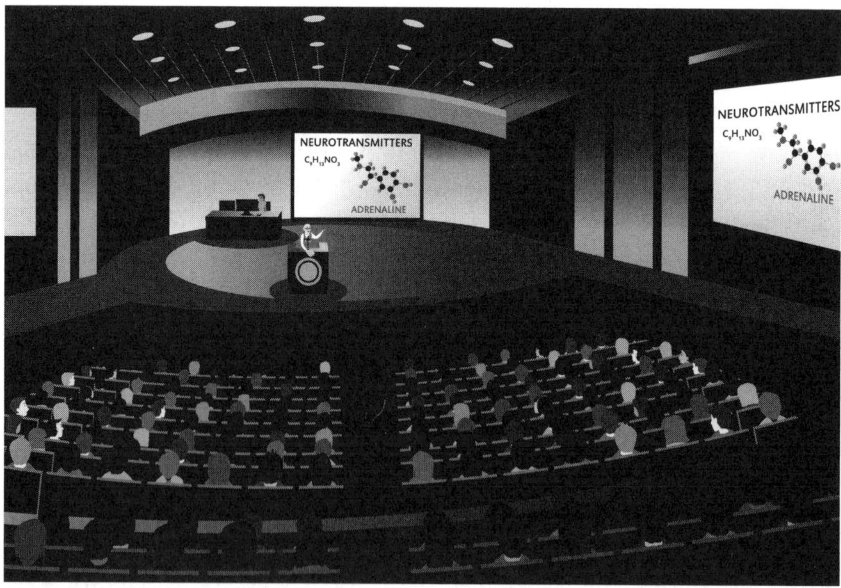

to teach classes in this way, knowing that it is not the best way for student learning to occur? It is my suggestion that we might be stuck within an old paradigm of the lecturing classroom. I am thankful that those reading this text are ready for a paradigm shift!

Students may also experience a loss of control with a change in teaching and learning methods within their classrooms. How many times have students asked, "Will this be on the test?" With a lecture, the students have a clear outline of what the faculty think are the most important issues. This leads students to an idea of what they are likely to be tested on. Could one extrapolate then, that lecture is a form of "teaching to the test"? When students are required to get out of their comfort zone and engage in their own learning, answer questions instead of ask them, create discussion rather than be a passive participant, they may feel a loss of control that they appreciate during a lecture. An active learning environment might be a bit uncomfortable at first, but is extremely engaging and fun for both the faculty and the students if given a chance.

Quast (2012) also believes resistance to change is a result of *bad timing*. In her opinion, loading too many changes on a person or group at one time will exponentially increase their resistance to change. However if change can be implemented slowly over time, the resistance tends to be less forceful. Resistance to change can also occur depending on the timing of the change itself. If a nurse educator is teaching a brand new course that is an all-new prep, it may not be a great time to try a new pedagogy. Too many changes all at once may result in failure. The timing of the implementation of the flipped classroom is therefore of utmost importance. Attempting to implement the flipped classroom method in the middle of an already-packed and busy semester is likely to add to an already challenging situation and result in an increase in faculty and student resistance. If nurse educators take their time to consider all the factors involved and use the advice in this text to help prepare themselves and their students, they are more likely to have a successful implementation. Proper timing cannot be understated.

We are all individuals with our own special personality traits. Resistance or acceptance to change fits into this preexisting personality. Quast (2012) would call this *an individual's predisposition toward change*. Some may prefer a set routine and become suspicious of change. Nurse educators with this type of mindset and personality are more likely to be resistant to any kind of proposed change, including the flipped classroom. On the other hand are those individuals that don't mind change at all. These nurse educators may enjoy a change because it brings about something new, fresh, and challenging. These types of people tend to be more flexible and able to go with the flow of the moment.

It would be fair to assume that the majority of nurse educators are naturally resistant to change and like to have more control of the classroom. So how can faculty and students be motivated to change the teaching and learning environment? A reflection over the past might reveal that the most challenging times also lead to transformation and successful change. Innovation does not occur without change, it is part of the definition. If we wish to be innovative nurse educators, we will need to face the uncertainty of change. I am challenging each nurse educator reading these pages to get out of the familiar comfort zone, and begin to see the possibilities of a new teaching and learning paradigm for nursing education. Considering the tidbits from Quast (2012) about how one might resist a change, and understanding individual personality and attitude about change, preparation for the changes of the flipped classroom seem more reasonable. A well-laid plan has the potential to remove many of the barriers to change that have been discussed.

Faculty Preparation for the Flipped Classroom

The first time I flipped the classroom, there was little research on the method in the available literature. Several studies about the flipped classroom have been reviewed in the text, but I am not sure that kind of evidence would have been very helpful to me the first time

I attempted the process. Most of the educational research studies had been done with smaller groups of students, not allowing for external validity. In addition, most of the more solid research findings were not within the profession of nursing. Most of the literature was anecdotal with little about how to actually implement the flipped classroom. To be honest, there was nothing available, even in hindsight, that would have helped me flip successfully without several strong hiccups along the way. Over the last several years of flipping the classroom, I have also come to realize that there are many different ways to flip a class. Every time I attend a flipping session at a conference or talk to a fellow nurse educator who is flipping their classroom, I realize the versatility of the pedagogy. The ability to flip virtually any nursing education content has brought about a variety of different approaches to flipping. Each faculty member can flip the classroom in his or her own unique way with a few steps of guidance along the way.

The next part of the chapter will provide some solid pearls of wisdom regarding faculty preparation for the flipped classroom. Some may seem almost elementary, but have proven to be some of the most important tidbits of information for faculty considering the flipped classroom.

Plan, Plan, and Then Plan Some More

In preparing for the process of flipping a classroom, *allow plenty of time to develop a solid plan*. The flipped classroom is not a pedagogy that faculty should run into without careful assessment and planning. The Intentional Instruction Model was designed for this particular purpose. Faculty who help students plan for theses or dissertations understand the importance of picking a due date and back tracking on the calendar with several small "goals" to get to the final product. Some of you may be writing a dissertation and thesis, and appreciate careful planning with the end in mind as well. The same concept can be used to create a timeline for flipping the classroom. The best advice would be to start the flipped classroom

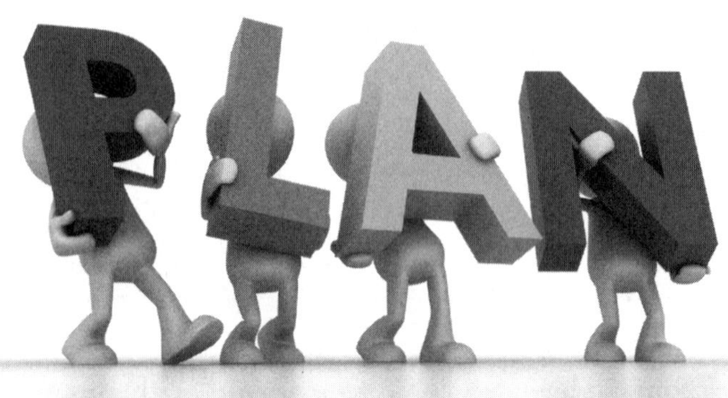

© CGinspiration/iStockPhoto

planning at least one semester or three calendar months prior to the time the flipped classroom will be implemented. Within this time frame a recording software of preference can be found and one can learn how to create and launch videos. This also affords adequate time to consider the best way to deliver the videos to students and time to plan the in-class activities and evaluation methods to match the predetermined learning objectives.

Planning for the flipped classroom should include both narrow-range and more expansive planning. The short-range planning should focus on the design for a certain class time. This planning includes pre-load and in-class activities as well as any associated evaluation methods. The more expansive planning should include the overarching strategies to achieve the objectives of the course. This bigger-picture plan may also include a curricular focus. As one might expect, it is difficult to do any of the more narrow-focused planning without first addressing the course and/or curricular planning. The following provides an example of the planning and how it may be accomplished.

Let's suppose it is May and Nursing Professor Susan wants to attempt flipping three classes within her upcoming physical assessment course in the fall. Her goal is to have everything ready to go by August 15 (the first day of classes). Working on a timeline, Susan can plan to do a little bit at a time over the next several weeks until she is prepared to implement her flipped classroom. **Figure 4-1** provides an example of how a timeline could be used to work on the flipped classroom one little piece at a time until the time to implement has arrived. Included with the timeline is a list of essential planning steps that can be used quite successfully. The time allotted for completion of each step really depends upon the individual nurse educator. Some may need to take a bit longer period of time to plan the different off-load and in-class objectives while others may need more time to learn the video software or find great videos and other content for the off-load portion. In general, it is recommended that one plan about 1 to 2 weeks for each of these steps. I have found that the most time-consuming part of flipping the classroom has been within the planning process. Taking time to ensure that the objectives match a flipped classroom may take some rewriting of original objectives and thoughtful planning. In the flipped classroom, the off-load objectives should be the lower-ordered objectives that students are likely to master on their own. Conversely, the in-class objectives are focused on higher-ordered learning so that the nurse educator can guide students into deeper understanding and comprehension of the material. Developing learning objectives in this manner allows for the best learning environments for students in both the off-load and in-class times available.

Planning for the evaluation piece of the puzzle may be a challenge, because some programs may have preset unchangeable evaluation pieces within the course and/or curriculum. For example, a Family Nurse Practitioner (FNP) course may use quite a bit of multiple-choice and write-in testing in order to prepare students for the experience of taking a certification examination. Similarly, in an undergraduate program multiple-choice testing may be a valued part of evaluation in order to prepare students for their board examination. However, there are some great ways to keep the multiple-choice–type quizzing and exams and also build in the idea of collaboration and referral. Group testing, allowing for a short collaboration period on 1 question, and the use of low-stakes quizzing with a classroom response system are some practical ideas.

1—Choose classes to flip 2—Get help	3—Learn software 4—Learning objectives	5—Redesign lecture 6 & 7—Test clip	8—Create Videos and launch	9—Develop in-class activities	10—Evaluation plan	11—Prep student plan	12—Launch	13—Evaluate
May 15th							Aug. 15th	

Flipped Classroom Planning To-Do List:

1. Pick 2 or 3 class periods that you feel comfortable flipping or whose objectives are particularly conducive to flipping.
2. Meet with an instructional designer and IT department if available to enlist help and advice.
3. Choose screen capture software and become familiar with how to use it.
4. Split learning objectives into lower and higher order using Bloom's Taxonomy.
5. Use lower-order objectives to craft or redesign lecture and cut back to 10–15 minutes of the *most pertinent* material in order to meet the off-load objectives.
6. Use software to record one slide or discussion point to test out the process.
7. Edit your short "test" clip and launch it to some kind of "test" audience.
8. Create final videos and find additional applicable off-load content for students prior to face-to-face class time.
9. Use higher order objectives to develop in class activities that match and augment the off-load content you've created for the students.
10. Create an evaluation plan for student learning and for evaluating your attempt at flipping.
11. Create a plan to prepare students for the flipped classroom.
12. Launch your flipped classroom.
13. Evaluate process and flipped classroom success or failure—revise plans within 1–2 weeks for next attempt at flipping this particular class.
14. Celebrate!

Figure 4-1 Timeline example.

Take It Slow and Proceed When Successful

The second most important advice is *don't take on too much at one time.* My first flipped classroom experience was with my good friend and colleague, Katherine (Kat) Johnson. We were so excited about the potential of the flipped classroom that we foolishly flipped the entire class and decided to do so a month prior to the class beginning. In hindsight, we now know that it would have been much smarter to flip one or two of our existing lecture-based classes to ease ourselves and our students into the flipped environment. We found the "all or nothing" approach to the flipped classroom to be too much for both students and faculty. We worked tirelessly that semester to get it right and attempted to make our students happier about the process. If we would have introduced the flipped classroom more slowly, we would have been able to assess our success and/or failure more gradually. Our students would have been gently eased into the change as well, instead of being pushed head first into the deep end of flipped learning.

Videos for the flipped classroom should be created, edited, and launched at least four days before class (for example, by Monday before a Thursday class), which means videos should be created, edited, loaded, tested, and ready to go the week prior to class. This gives students plenty of time to fit them into their existing schedules. With students who are busy with their work, family/social lives, and often are taking other classes at the same time they are taking the flipped classroom course(s), it is only fair to give them several days of time prior to class to watch the videos. This approach is more successful than posting the videos the night before class and expecting students to watch them and be prepared for in-class activities.

There are several classes to flip, so which one should you choose? There are a couple of ways you can make this choice. You may already have in mind one or two classes that would be particularly conducive to the flipped classroom. A class that has learning objectives with many higher-ordered skills would be a good place to start. These classes are likely to be complex, and the students could use the expertise of the nursing faculty as a guide for student learning as they practice more hands-on or higher-ordered skill development. For example, in a FNP course the suturing class and the class focusing on X-ray interpretation could easily be flipped. For the suturing class, a short video can be provided on the basics of suturing with information such as what types of sutures to use for which types of wounds, basic wound management and asepsis, how long stitches need to be in place, and so on. The entire in-class time can then be used to work on the types of stitches and use of the suturing equipment. Similarly, the X-ray class could provide off-load material including the basics of what to order and why, differences between CT and MRI, and a couple of basic interpretation pearls. When the students get to class, the time is spent reviewing several X-ray examples and working together to do a wet read. Class time could also be spent on case studies of how a patient might present with injury and what type of imaging study should be ordered and why. When students have completed classes such as these, there is an additional advantage of the videos to provide a review and to solidify what they learned in class. Knowing that these students will be tested on content, some mock quizzing

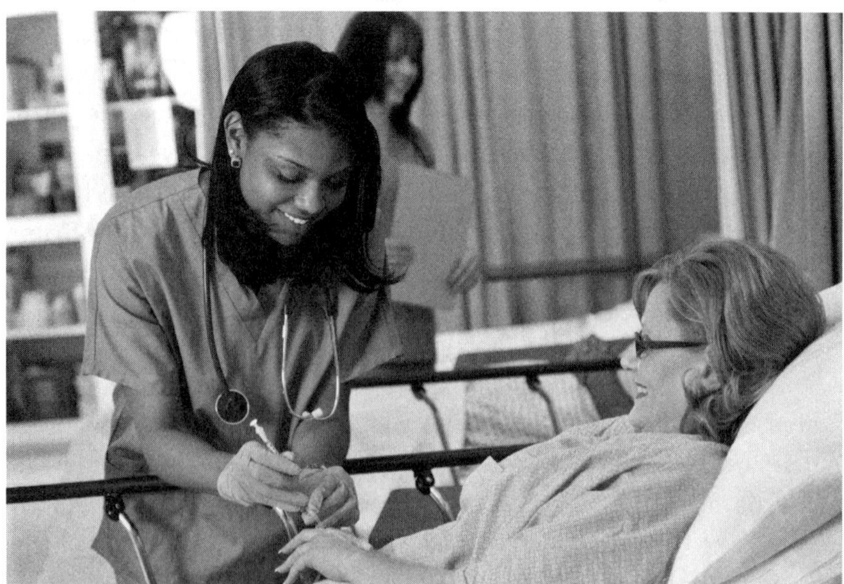

© Steve Debenport/iStockPhoto

during the class time to give students an idea of what types of quiz questions might be on an upcoming test can alleviate student anxiety with active learning in comparison to a lecture-only pedagogy.

Many tend to think of using one's hands when they hear the word "skill." However, the term *skill* can also be used in the sense of critical thinking and knowledge application rather than just knowledge acquisition. For example, many FNP courses have a great number of higher-order application objectives as the program prepares students to make diagnostic and treatment decisions based on a set of possible diagnoses called *differential diagnoses*. Such critical thinking is very high ordered and students often have a difficult time sifting through all of the many factors that could be associated with a diagnosis and treatment plan. In this setting, the use of problem-based and case-based learning to accomplish higher-ordered thinking and application of material can be positive teaching and learning strategies. Problem-based learning (PBL) is a student-centered, inquiry-based pedagogy approach that helps students discover their own solutions to real-life problems through either individual or cooperative group work (Oja, 2011). In his review, Oja found that even though there have been different approaches to PBL in the nursing education research literature, it has been shown to improve critical thinking in nursing students.

Case-based learning is very similar, but focuses the problem-based learning on a specific case study. In Spain, Raurell-Torreda and colleagues (2014) conducted a nonrandomized controlled trial with comparison of clinical skills between groups of students who had been exposed to case-based learning and those who had not. They found that the intervention group did develop better patient assessment skills in their undergraduate nursing student sample. The researchers theorized that improving sets of skills using case-based learning is similar to putting the student into a virtual clinical environment with a patient who is in need of their care. Doing so requires decision making and complex analysis of disease process, culture, developmental age/stage, and so on. Working within Benner's Novice

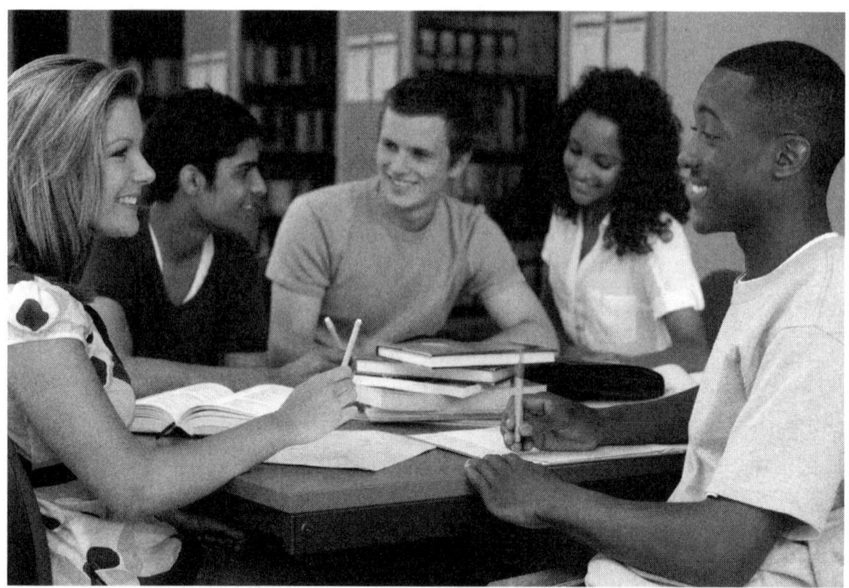

to Expert theory (2001), these types of virtual case-based learning experiences can prepare students for real clinical encounters. Each time student are presented with a case-based patient, they can practice patient cares and interventions with the guidance of their expert faculty member at their side. In group work settings, they also learn the art of collaboration and decision making within a group of colleagues rather than on their own. The in-class portion of the text will provide more information on how to develop this type of learning opportunity within the classroom.

When deciding which classes to flip, it is also recommended that faculty choose topics they feel the most confident in teaching. When flipping the classroom, the faculty are taking themselves out of the driver's seat within the classroom. When this happens, there is more of a chance for divergent learning and expanded learning that moves past the original learning objectives. When this occurs, faculty may feel most comfortable when they have professional experience with the subject matter within their own clinical past. For example,

I would be more hesitant to flip a class focused on genetics. I think the field of genetics is fascinating, but I have not had personal experience with this topic. It is very likely that the students will ask me questions that I will not be able to answer. Although I don't think that this scenario is a bad one at all, I do think that when you are focused on attempting to flip the classroom for the first time, it would create less pressure to choose a subject or class that you are confident in discussing and expanding student knowledge from your own experience. I would, however, have no problem discussing quite deeply a labor and delivery case study or one focused on high-risk outpatient obstetrical care because I have a great deal of professional clinical experience from which to draw. It is definitely not a hard-and-fast rule, but faculty might feel less pressure with a first attempt at the flipped classroom environment if they are able to teach "on the fly."

There are numerous occasions that I look things up with students, even when I do know the answer. As I mentioned previously, I do not think that this is bad practice. We are modeling for our students the spirit of evidence-based practice and helping them to understand where and how to find the most accurate and up-to-date information. But when attempting to flip the classroom initially, it would be easier to choose topics that you could teach with your eyes closed and both hands tied behind your back. You will also have more ideas for off-load and in-class materials for those topics you feel most comfortable with. The clinical or personal professional experience that faculty have with a certain subject provides a virtual untapped gold mine of learning activities for the in-class session. More of how to use these experiences within your flipped classroom will be explored in coming chapters.

Once nurse educators flip the classroom, they should be certain to spend a bit of reflective time on what worked and what did not. Even if the educators feel like everything went really well in their flipped classroom, they should think about how they could do it better, use time more efficiently, and engage every student every minute of the class. It can become a personal challenge to get better each and every time a flipped class is conducted. After the nurse educator has successfully flipped two or three of classes, it is time to proceed! The average semester consists of about 16 weeks of material if not in a blocked session. If the flipped classroom is used in two or three of the classes each semester, the educator will have half or more of the class flipped with success by the third or fourth go round. Although this may seem like a slow process, it will make a great deal of difference toward success with the pedagogy. In addition, the students will be able to hold onto their occasional lecture with interactivity while they are getting used to the flipped classroom. They will be eased into the method and hopefully begin to see the benefit of the method to their learning. Lastly, this slow progression of change with the same group of students may lend itself to a nice research study assessing the success and adoption of the method by students.

Get Help

All have most likely heard the saying, "Rome wasn't built in a day." Well, it wasn't built by one person, either! Not only should the planning begin well in advance of the flipping date of implementation, but faculty should also *engage all of the help and assistance that is available!* Some instructors consider themselves tech savvy and won't use information technology (IT) assistance that is available. I tend to be this type of faculty member, quick to click on links, try programs out for myself and ask the questions later. Who has time to find out before clicking? Well, this is one aspect of flipping that I can provide some valuable advice from experience. This "can do" attitude often turns into a "could've done better" attitude in hindsight. I was in such a hurry to flip the classroom that I didn't even take the time to watch the instructional videos for the screen capture software I was using. Although they were readily available on my campus, I never attended a faculty session on how to operate the software, either. In hindsight, this was a major mistake. I still managed to create videos and at a fairly high quality, but it took me a long, long time to do so. About a year later, I attended a session on how to use the software correctly. I was surprised to find out how much I didn't know about the program, the quick and easy shortcuts, and the excellent features such as editing that I could have used when recording and editing my videos. It seems like such a simple piece of advice, but faculty who learn to use the screen capture software fully prior to attempting to use it will save valuable time and decrease frustration.

Developing Lecture Videos

Tying in with the idea of seeking out help from an IT crew and/or viewing instructional videos on screen capture software, start by making 2- to 3-minute video clips that are meaningless. These small clips will allow practice using the software. In addition to creating these little clips, try launching them to test out that process as well.

The first time I made a video, I did not think about these simple steps. I had the lecture slides from a past lecture, sat down at the computer, and started to record. I filled a video with 45 minutes (this is way too long, by the way) full of useful information I would have provided for lecture if students were sitting in their classroom seats in front of me. Feeling proud of myself for my technologically savvy mind, I opened the video editing part of the program to review my last hour of work. . .finding that I had recorded no audio whatsoever. What a waste of time! Going back into my computer sound mixer, I found that I had the audio muted the entire time. Here is just one example of how accessing the "how-to" videos for the software would have saved me valuable time. It also provides support for recording a one- or two-slide portion of your presentation to see if you are doing everything correctly. I promise that the 3 minutes of time it takes to practice with the software will save you an hour or more of frustration!

Once the video had been recorded (with sound this time), I began to play with the editing abilities within the screen capture software. I love to play with editing features, and spent way too much time on my first videos putting in beautiful title pages, transition after wonderful transition between the slides, call-outs to make my points, and so on. I can remember taking about 30 minutes of time on one little section of a video, making sure the call-out box I had added came in and left just the way I wanted it to. I think I am either too much of a perfectionist or just in need some good, solid counseling. I have learned my lesson, and now when I record a video, I leave out all the fancy bells and whistles and just produce the video as is. The students have told me that they do not care about all the "pretty" things on the video, they only care that I am talking to them and telling them what they need to know to be prepared for in-class activities. The take-home point is to not be distracted by attempting to make the videos fancy or entertaining. It takes up way too much time and does not make any difference to your target audience in the long run.

Other fellow flipping professors have told me that their students prefer videos made by the professor they will be seeing in class. They would rather not watch a video made by someone else that can be found on the Internet; they actually prefer listening to their own instructors! This is such a wonderful surprise, because most of us despise the sound of our own voice on the videos. The discomfort with our own voice and video within a picture-in-picture are things we need to put aside. Our students like the videos better when they are made by the faculty teaching the course. There is no doubt that a similar professionally made video could be found on the Internet with the many educational websites now available. But students have voiced that they feel more connected to their own faculty and want to learn from their lecture videos, have access to their special views, experiences, and touch on the content that is being discussed within the video. So to reiterate, try to avoid getting caught up in all of the editing features when making videos. The video you make will be just right for your students' needs. Let's face it, we are not movie producers, we are educators. Lastly, try to set aside the discomfort of not liking the sound of your own voice on the video. Remember that students prefer your voice on the videos and they are not interested in additional formatting that might make our videos seem more professional. Keep it simple.

Launching Your Lecture Videos

Once you have expertly created your video, you have to give the students access to it. There are a variety of ways this can be done, but once again, plan and practice this step plenty of time in advance.

After my first video was created, I launched it to the YouTube account that I had created for the purpose of the flipped classroom. Not wanting anyone else to hear by voice and have access to my "treasure," I chose the box labeled "private." Yes, I want this to be private, I said to myself and I launched it into the Internet abyss. Next was the email to the students letting them know that their first video was available for them to view. The link to the video was provided within the email. Job well done, I thought to myself, and went to bed.

I would soon regret choosing the little box "private," because several harsh comments from my students started pouring into my email box the next day. I know that some of you are smiling at this point, understanding that when you choose to make a video private, you must invite every single person you want to view that video by providing their email on the website. In addition, each person who wants to view the video needs to have an active Google account. At this point in time, this is not such a big deal, because many of our students have an account anyway, but it is not something I had planned on or prepared them for.

The students unfortunately took this "rookie" mistake to the bank, and refused to attempt to access any additional link I had sent them to watch the video. Now, rewind about 2 weeks and imagine if I had taken my own advice and launched the video ahead of time, inviting a friend, previous student I trust, or fellow faculty to view the video. I would have found out long before that I needed to choose "unlisted" and not "private" when I launched the video. I cannot stress enough how valuable taking time to test things out ahead of time will be to your flipping classroom success story.

Consider Flipping With a Colleague or Group of Colleagues

I feel like my colleague Kat and I working through our first experience of flipping the classroom together made it a more enjoyable endeavor. We were able to encourage one another and help each other when needed. We also found that working together allowed us to share ideas for both videos and in-class activities that worked well for each of us. Using those ideas, we morphed them into our own subject matter and were able to come up with several great interactive learning activities for our students during the class time. I think that the only better scenario would have been for us to have been in the classroom together during the in-class learning portion of the flipped classroom. Instead, I taught my half of the class at the beginning of the semester, and then Kat came in to teach her half during the second part of the semester. Being there to help each other during the in-class time would have made it easier on both of us. Most in-class activities require faculty to circulate and interact with students around the room. Having two of us to interact with students would have been a better idea, in hindsight. It would be my suggestion to work with someone else who has similar expertise or see if employing a graduate teaching assistant is possible. This approach has the potential to make the in-class portion a bit less taxing and allow for sharing of ideas. Graduate assistants provide an excellent second expert during the in-class session, and have the additional benefit of learning about teaching along the way.

Completing videos with another faculty member or content expert has also been suggested. Developing a video with another instructor allows for you to "play off of" one another, and ask questions that a student might ask. It also allows for a more stimulating video for your students, because two voices are more entertaining and interesting than one. I have not been able to create videos with another faculty member yet, but this is definitely on my flipping "to-do" list. An additional idea I have is to take this idea one step further and ask a student to join me for the taping of the video. There are always a few really engaged students who ask excellent questions that could be enlisted in this type of team video. It might be better to ask students who have already completed the course rather than those who are currently taking the course. I have mentioned this idea to a group of students in the past and several thought it was a brilliant idea. They also mentioned that they would be able to play that "student" role very well, and perhaps add into the video some examples of how they learned the material or were able to study more effectively in order to pass an exam successfully. For example, one student mentioned his ability to create easy acronyms and analogies for learning concepts in order to prepare for classes and exams that he would like to share with his fellow students. I love the idea of enlisting students to help students in the videos. I wish I had more information for you on whether it is a success or not. One thing is certain, students seem to be interested in helping their fellow students learn—another advantage of the flipped classroom model.

To help prepare for the flipped classroom, consider finding a group of faculty that are planning to flip the classroom during the same period of time. I had the great privilege to work with a group of professors across campus on the intricacies of the flipped classroom called The Flipped Learning Academy. Having a provost who is very interested in innovation, technology, and pedagogy best practices, The Flipped Learning Academy was designed to educate and support faculty from across disciplines interested in the flipped classroom pedagogy. The biggest benefit of being a part of this type of group was the conversation with fellow faculty members. There were faculty involved from all kinds of programs across campus, such as nutrition, nursing, mathematics, biology, philosophy, and speech and language pathology, to name just a few. Sharing conversation and discussion time with these great minds, dissecting ideas about the flipped classroom, and sharing individual successes and failures with pedagogy in general has proven to be extremely helpful. It is highly recommended that nursing faculty interested in flipping the classroom find a similar group. Sharing ideas with other faculty is a most valuable and helpful approach to flipping, whether one is a seasoned educator or a novice faculty member teaching a course for the first time.

Organizing the Learning Objectives

As depicted within the Intentional Instruction Model, everything developed for the flipped classroom should flow from the existing learning objectives. If possible, it would be ideal to develop the learning objectives with the flipped classroom in mind. Either way, it will be important to take some time to organize the learning objectives for each class into lower- and higher-ordered objectives. Those that fit into the lower-level objectives can be accomplished with the off-load materials, while those higher-ordered objectives can be addressed in the live class with the student and instructor working together. The Bloom's stair step developed by Patty Shank (2013) is very helpful to organize these objectives and think about some of the teaching strategies that are conducive for each (**Figure 4-2**).

The stairs in the model show the lower-level objective terms at the bottom of the stair case, which increase with each additional stair

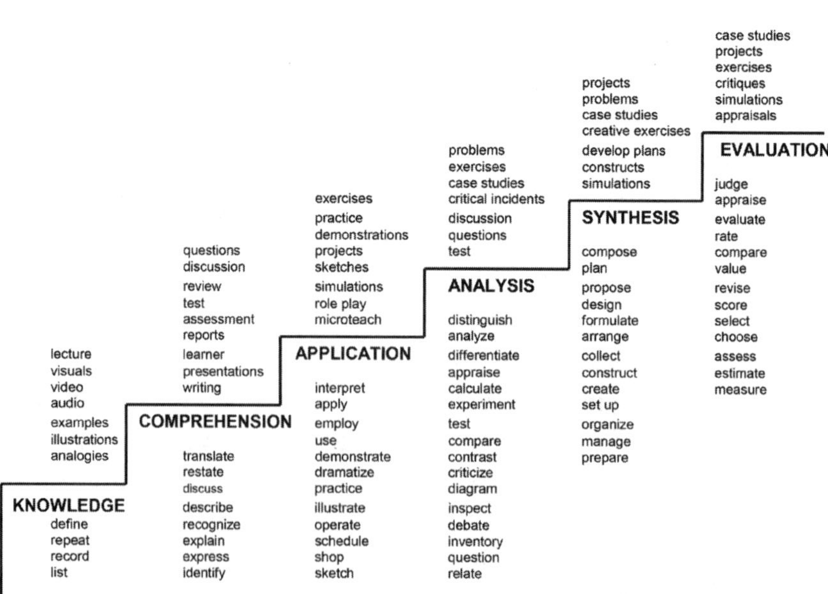

Figure 4-2 Bloom's stair step.
Natural Resources Conservation Service

climbed. I understand that a lengthy discussion about how to write learning objectives is not necessary within the pages of this text. However, organizing the learning objectives to match the different facets of the flipped classroom is necessary. You may even find that you may need to rewrite some learning objectives for each class to more readily match the capability of the flipped classroom. It has been a nice surprise to see how much higher on the Bloom's ladder students can climb when the flipped classroom is applied.

Give Yourself a Break!

Nursing faculty and graduate nursing students tend to hold themselves to a very high standard in general. Nursing faculty and graduate students studying to be future faculty are likely to want to be as close to perfection as possible. It is necessary to remind current and future faculty to not be too hard on themselves. The flipped classroom is a pedagogy that takes some time to master. A fear is that instant perfection and/or success with the method will turn some faculty away from the method altogether. Some flipping attempts are just better than others. Some flipping classes work really well with one group of students and end up bombing with another group. There are so many variables that can affect the teaching and learning atmosphere. Taking time to try the method and revise it until success is achieved takes some perseverance for sure. Try not to be too hard on yourself and realize that this is a learning curve that may take a little time to perfect. I want your flipping experience to be something positive. For that to occur, we might have to accept the fact that things might not go the way we thought they would or should. It does not make the attempt a failure. Failure would be not trying anything new at all and staying within a pedagogical shell for the rest of one's nursing education career. Take it easy on yourself and allow for some error to occur. It is natural. It is sometimes the best way we can learn how to do things in a better or more efficient way.

Within this same line of thought is the concept of letting the little things go. I recall very vividly a conversation with a young and extremely intelligent instructor flipping her class. She mentioned struggling with a particular student who was adamant about not engaging in the concept of the flipped classroom. She had 99% of her students engaged and loving the flipped classroom. She was successful in every other way, but this one student would not submit and continued to give her a hard time over the instructional method. She was not sure how to win the student over, and we spent some time discussing the issue. It dawned on me that making everyone happy all the time is not realistic, but it doesn't stop this from being our goal. We discussed a few strategies on how to "win over" this one student, but in the end I think what this brilliant young educator needed was some validation that she was working hard to teach the material, and that flipping was working for 99% of her students. It reminded me of when I read my student evaluations at the end of each semester. I generally receive fairly high teaching scores and positive student comments, but there is always one student who didn't like my teaching for one reason or another. I have to let this go and realize that it is possible to make some of the people happy some of the time, but not everyone happy all of the time. We will have some students who might not not agree with the pedagogy of the flipped classroom. There is much we can do to prepare them, but there will still be some that do not like this teaching style or the way the material is delivered. I take comfort in knowing that not all of the students liked the way I taught when I used straight lecture either. But bad reviews continue to be difficult to swallow. The upcoming chapter on preparing the students for flipped learning can help with the expected resistance, but it may still exist. Don't be too hard on yourself and don't forget to celebrate your successes along the way.

References

Benner, P. (2001). *From novice to expert: Excellence and power in clinical nursing practice.* New Jersey: Prentice-Hall.

Halvorson, J. G. (2012). *Explained: Why we don't like change.* Retrieved from http://www.huffingtonpost.com/heidi-grant-halvorson-phd/why-we-dont-like-change_b_1072702.html

Oja, K. J. (2011). Using problem-based learning in the clinical setting to improve nursing students' critical thinking: An evidence review. *Journal of Nursing Education, 50*(3), 145–151.

Prensky, M. (2010). *Teaching digital natives: Partnering for real learning.* Thousand Oaks, CA: Sage.

Quast, L. (2012). *Overcome the 5 main reasons people resist change.* Retrieved from http://www.forbes.com/sites/lisaquast/2012/11/26/overcome-the-5-main-reasons-people-resist-change/

Raurell-Torreda, M., Olivet-Pujol, J., Romero-Collado, A., Malagon-Aguilera, M. C., Patino-Maso, J., & Baltasar-Bague, A. (2014). Case-based learning and simulation: Useful tools to enhance nurses' education? Nonrandomized controlled trial. *Journal of Nursing Education and Scholarship, 41*(1), 34–42.

Shank, P. (2013). *e-Learning guild: Reconsidering Bloom's taxonomy (old and new).* Retrieved from http://www.learningsolutionsmag.com/articles/1105/

CHAPTER 5

Preparing Your Students for the Flipped Classroom

Students and the Flipped Classroom

Students and faculty may share some resistance to the flipped classroom for many of the same reasons. It is no surprise that students have the potential to experience a certain amount of discomfort with the new pedagogy. In order for the flipped classroom to be successful, *a paradigm shift of teaching and learning* is required of *both* students and faculty. More work and engagement will be required of everyone involved in the teaching and learning atmosphere as the flipped classroom is implemented. Students who have been exposed to a classroom with any type of interactive learning method find that it requires more attention and work on their part. If they are not ready or invested in this change, they are likely to be resistant to it.

The previous chapter focused on how to prepare faculty for the flipped classroom. Now it is time to turn that attention to preparing students for the flipped classroom. Just as there are two sides to the teaching and learning dyad, there are two parties involved in the flipped classroom preparation process. Both parties will be experiencing the changes associated with the flipped classroom. Preparing oneself as a faculty member will not be enough. There must also be a solid plan created to prepare students for the change that they are being asked to be a part of.

How Do We Engage Our Students?

When developing the first rendition of the Intentional Instruction Model, it was clear that the students had been left out of the picture. Students may not be inspired and be automatically engaged to learn just because nurse educators want them to. The fact that a tuition-paying student is not always ready to learn is counterintuitive, but a reality in higher education. Nurse educators are fortunate that the majority of nursing students are interested in learning how to be a nurse. The future work of the student is dependent upon the education they are receiving, and that is a huge advantage in terms of student engagement in the classroom. The information in this chapter is focused on students who may question or be uncomfortable with new pedagogy in their classroom. Although it seems to imply that all students are difficult or resistant, that is not the intention of the chapter. Most students are open to new teaching and learning strategies and have a terrific attitude about their individual learning. There are, however, those instances when students do show less enthusiasm and willingness to be a part of new pedagogical approaches. The chapter is focused on how to prepare all students toward the goal of informing and partnering with them rather than dictating what the classroom atmosphere will be for the semester.

Consider a possible scenario to begin the discussion of student learning and retaining of information from one nursing course to another. Imagine the nurse educator spent a great deal of time teaching a topic to a group of students only to find that they performed poorly on an associated exam. Or perhaps there has been a conversation between faculty members who are teaching content that builds from one semester to the next. One faculty member might voice frustration due to the students not learning content that was to be taught in a past course that they needed in order to understand the content in their current course. A more specific example might sound familiar. Faculty teaching the pediatrics content became concerned that the students didn't know what a peak flow reading was or how to obtain one. The peak flow and associated meaning and skills had been taught in the curriculum three times prior to the students taking the pediatrics course. Some faculty may relate to this scenario, in which they were sure that the students had a good understanding of a concept or skill, only to find out that they did not retain that information for future coursework in the program. It might be that even the most skilled nurse educators find that students have a difficult time retaining some information taught to them, even when hands-on skills are an associated part of the teaching and learning process.

The scenario above certainly brings about a confusing and frustrating dilemma. These types of scenarios happening to a young faculty member or graduate student aspiring to be an educator might bring the realization that there is a definite difference between *teaching* and *learning*. Even when nursing faculty are sure that they've taught the content well, students may have difficulty retaining the content for future recall and use. Those more experienced educators may not be as surprised by this educational disconnect. Some might even claim that there is a phenomenon called "brain dump" where the students forget content naturally after the semester is over. Nursing students need to be able to build knowledge upon knowledge and apply that to the care of patients. Therefore, the theory of a "brain dump" does not seem like a plausible explanation for why students might not retain information taught. Perhaps the problem of retaining important content from semester to semester has more to do with the way in which students learn and are honored as an important part of the teaching and learning dyad.

Cognitive load theory (Swellar, van Merrienboer, & Pass, 1998) posits that for learning to occur, students should have stored learned information into their long-term memory. Once stored or learned, that information should be available for rapid recall when necessary (such as in a future pediatrics course). If students are not able to recall information from their long-term memory for a future course, perhaps learning had not occurred in the previous course. So why discuss cognitive load theory, student brain architecture, and student motivation to learn? Well, the students must be willing and able to *learn* what nurse educators are teaching. To be able to teach the students, nurse educators must work together with nursing students in a fluid teaching and learning team. Each member of this team has a certain amount of responsibility to the way in which teaching is conducted and learning is assimilated. What can we learn about the relationship between instructor and student or a group of students?

Relationship in Teaching and Learning

Many might agree that teaching and learning are fluid concepts, not different entities. Within a classroom or clinical setting, it could be argued that the faculty member is teaching and the students are learning. There could also be a situation in which the student is teaching and the faculty are learning. It is well known that there is a scenario in which students teach each other. Students in study groups have been shown to be more successful than those who study alone (Hendry, Hyde, & Davy, 2005). Each of these dimensions can occur at different times within the teaching and learning landscape, which allows for a deeply rich and valuable set of experiences for student learning. In nursing education classrooms that only use lecture, only one dimension of learning mentioned above is allowed. The flipped classroom allows for students to take a more active role not only in their own learning, but an active role in teaching one another as well. Our students will be doing a great deal of teaching when they are in their graduated clinical roles, whether that be as a registered nurse, advanced practice nurse, or nurse educator. The ability to practice teaching others is a valuable skill that is allowed within the flipped classroom model.

Each educator or graduate student reading these pages can most likely recall times that they've learned from their students or student colleagues. Students can teach us new things if they are given the chance. This is one reason being a nurse educator is so wonderful. What students teach faculty or each other may be very small, but have a big impact. For example, some students have taken the time to teach me about their culture, or a different perspective that they share. Sometimes what is learned is more concrete, such as a certain way to combine medications to enhance the quality of care that they learned from their preceptor in clinical. In reality, our students are our future colleagues. When nurse educators approach their students with this type of paradigm, they may begin to see them differently. Instead of seeing the students as empty vessels that must be filled with information, they are viewed as knowledgeable and highly capable individuals who need a little mentoring and coaching. Each student is someone we may work beside in the future. Our current student could be the nurse who will be assigned to take care of one of our family members or ourselves someday in their clinical settings. Students not only have great potential, but also possess current professional worth. Allowing sharing of ideas, reciprocal learning, and collaboration may foster a collegial approach to problem solving in nursing student groups.

With this approach to teaching future colleagues, a mutual working relationship with students can flourish in nursing education classrooms and clinical settings. Perhaps Bergmann and Sams say it best, "good teaching has always been about relationship" (2014, p. 21). They go on to state, "The relationship that a teacher develops with his or her students is what makes teaching good regardless of whether or not a teacher flips a class" (2014, p. 21). Bergmann and Sams propose that the content, although central to learning and important in terms of curriculum, should not take up 90% of the educational picture, leaving relationship and student curiosity to fight over the last 10%. Instead, they envision content, curiosity, and relationship sharing the picture, each having an equal one-third of the educational "pie," if you will. Prensky (2010) agrees that as educators we need to put the focus on people and their passions rather than classes and content. In his work on partnering with students, he discusses "passion-based learning" in which students are asked what they are passionate about on an individual rather than a group basis. Prensky believes that taking the time to discover what each student is passionate about will help them as the student and you as the educator. With this type of relationship, we can begin to understand how a student's passion is connected to who they are, and be able to motivate them to learn on a different level.

Bergmann and Sams make such a valuable point about K-12 education that we share in nursing education. Many curricula are too large, too specific, and offer too little flexibility for student exploration. Educators should be intentional about what they offer the students as content, using content as a "conduit to teach the process of learning and to instill a passion for knowledge" (2014, p. 23) in their students. Would it be feasible to do this in nursing education? Can we leave room for student self-discovery, passion, and exploration of content?

> *"When done well, teaching is fundamentally a human interaction in which the passions and interest of the students are fanned to a flame."*
>
> (Bergmann & Sams, 2014, p. 26)

Can We Leave Room for Student Curiosity?

Bergmann and Sams (2014) go on to discuss the curiosity that a student brings to the educational setting. Students have questions! They are curious and want to learn. It was a surprise for me to see that Bergmann and Sams were discussing the same curricular overload in K-12 education that we are experiencing in nursing education. Teachers in both settings just have too much content to cover. Due to this, educators may be hesitant to allow student choice in what to learn or how they wish to go about learning. What we teach has been determined over the years by our accrediting agencies, which are made up of several content experts in the field of nursing. It was interesting to learn that Bergmann and Sams have both served on similar curricular committees and found that each expert believed their area of content to be the most important and essential to include. The result was a bloated curriculum that could not possibly be delivered within the expected time frame. Content experts have had years and years of experience in their chosen field. Can we ever hope to teach students to this type of expert level in their nursing programs? It may not be realistic to think we can keep adding content to programs but never change the way the content is taught to or delivered to the students from a teaching and learning perspective. One might also ask if individual student curiosity can play into this curricular picture, or does it?

I recently went to a presentation on the concept-based curriculum at the University of Nebraska Medical Center on the Western Campus by Dr. Susan Wilhelm and Dr. Teresa Rodehorst-Weber, two of my favorite undergraduate nursing instructors. I was fascinated to hear them talk about letting go of their expert-based curriculum in exchange for a curriculum that was focused on teaching the students basics for entry into practice as a registered nurse. I began to feel myself cringe a bit, as they described how they took specialty courses like pediatrics and obstetrics out of the curriculum as separate courses. Although the idea made sense, I could not help but feel a loss due to my own personal love of obstetric nursing. It would seem that my 20 years of experience with this population should be of use, and taught to every single student in an undergraduate nursing program. The fact of the matter is that the curriculum did not leave out obstetrics or pediatrics. Instead, the curriculum was approaching education of nurses from a more practical framework.

As they described how nursing curricula had become saturated with more and more content over the years and how they came to the realization that they had to let go of their expert mindset and began to think about nursing education in terms of entry level into practice, it resonated with me. They discussed teaching the students how to learn and gain new knowledge on their own, which I loved and completely agree with. Their approach is an exemplar for nursing education that echoes the ideas of Bergmann and Sams (2014) to instill and encourage curiosity in our students. But when it is all said and done in both K-12 and higher education, students really have little choice in what and how they want to learn.

Could we begin to give students a portion of their learning time to explore their own interests within the flipped classroom model? Bergmann and Sams (2014) say *yes*! Because of the class time that is freed by moving lecture to a home-based learning tool, they are describing what some teachers are calling "Genius Hour" or the "20% time" (2014, p. 25). Within this time, students are given about 20% of the class time to work on passion-based projects and research. They do so with guidance from the instructor, and are required to demonstrate their learning in a variety of ways. The point is that students get to choose what they want to learn, how they want to learn it, and what type of learning outcome they prefer. Although I have not been able to experiment with the 20% time yet, it is something I am planning to implement in my courses. It is a strategy that allows for more partnering with student groups and a way to gain their support of the flipped classroom, as well.

The ideas of individualized learning and partnering with students when initiating the flipped classroom make a lot of good sense. These approaches help us to strategize for ultimate student investment in the flipped classroom, and their adoption of it as a new and different approach to their learning. Tying together the concepts of Bergmann and Sams (2014), Prensky (2010), and Kotter's Process for Leading Change (Kotter, 2015), nursing faculty can develop a solid plan to prepare their students for the flipped classroom. A review of each of Kotter's 8 steps will follow, each with an application to the nursing education classroom.

Kotter's 8-Step Process for Leading Change

According to the 40 years of research by Dr. John Kotter, more than 70% of all transformation efforts in organizations fail due to the lack of a consistent approach to change and engaging the workforce in the change efforts (Kotter, 2015). I will confess that the first time I flipped the classroom, I was part of this 70% failure for a couple of reasons. The first was that I had no consistent plan or approach to this change for myself or my students. Instead, I assumed the students would "fall in line" with my new ideas without any questioning or resistance at all. I also did not include my students (known as the *workforce* in Kotter's work) in the process of the educational change.

According to Kotter (2015), the organizations that have been successful with change efforts tend to have the same 3 characteristics in common. First of all, they followed a change process closely and paid attention to factors of change, including the anticipatory guidance a model can provide. Secondly, they allowed the process to be flexible and apply to their specific needs and contexts. Thirdly, they measured their change efforts in terms of their results or outcomes (Kotter, 2015). We are in a perfect position to employ all three of these "success steps" as we prepare ourselves and our students for any major educational change.

Step 1: Create a Sense of Urgency

The first step of Kotter's 8-step Process for Leading Change (**Figure 5-1**) is *Create a Sense of Urgency*. Kotter describes this as "crafting and using a significant opportunity as a means for exciting people to sign up to change their organization" (Kotter, 2015).

For nursing instructors, I like to think that this is an easy step. In nursing education, we are fortunate that the content matter that we are teaching is directly connected to our students' ability to function in their desired role as a nurse. Even before they graduate, they must apply the principles and approaches to patient care that they have learned in the classrooms within their clinical settings. If they are not ready and prepared, a patient could be injured or even die. We work within a clinical profession that requires us to make decisions that can affect the life or death of a patient. This one fact should be motivating enough for our students to create a sense of urgency.

I remember as a nursing student the anxiety of realizing that my actions have very definite consequences in the real world of nursing care. What I did as the nurse could be the difference between my

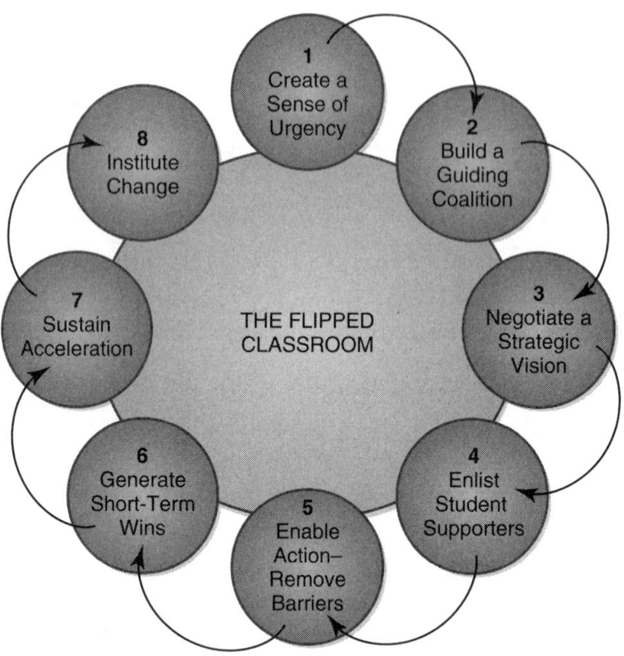

Figure 5-1 Kotter's change model applied to the flipped classroom.
Modified from http://www.kotterinternational.com/the-8-step-process-for-leading-change/

patient going home to their family members or going to the graveyard. I actually still cannot think about this too much because it can be paralyzing to me as a provider. The good news is that this jewel of motivation is perfect to create an atmosphere of urgency to learn how to do things correctly. Suddenly the coursework is not so much about getting the best grade or being the best student. It is about taking care of patients the most effective and safe way we possibly can.

I was fortunate enough to have Jean Watson as my philosophy of science professor during my PhD education at the University of Colorado Health Sciences Center. What a treat that was. It is really something to be in the presence of greatness. When discussing Dr. Watson's Theory of Human Caring in particular, one student in the course with a very high-powered personality who worked all of her life in the emergency room. She brought up a valid but bold point to the well-known theorist. She asked Dr. Watson about her theory as it would apply to her ER setting, postulating that caring theory was fine for some areas of nursing, but could not possibly apply to her "unique" ER environment. The calm and thoughtful response from Dr. Watson was that the very fact that the ER nurse studies and learns how to take care of the emergent patient with ease and efficiently shows his/her caring attitude. Why else would the ER nurse learn how to take care of these patients so successfully? The response allows us to see that caring attitude may show up a little differently for different nursing professionals. The sense of urgency to care for patients correctly is directly connected to a caring attitude toward any patient population. The students understand and can relate to this story when thinking about their motivation to learn safe and quality patient care to the best of their ability. Caring demeanor can create a sense of urgency to learn nursing content.

Creating a sense of urgency for students can look different depending on the topics of the course. For example, creating a sense of urgency to know how to treat a patient who is in a hypertensive crisis quickly and effectively is a great motivator. We can impress upon the students that they need to be prepared in this type of emergency in order to save a life. When we are teaching nursing theory or research method, the urgency is a bit harder to generate. However, I have found through my experiences as a nursing educator that the more applicable I can make the content to the nursing care work the students will be engaged in, they have more interest in learning the material. I have also learned that allowing them to apply the material in a way that is meaningful to them is very helpful. Here we touch again on Prensky's (2010) and Bergmann and Sams' (2014) concepts of allowing for individualization and student curiosity.

If I assign a nursing theory to students and make them apply it to hypertension, they may not be as engaged and interested as if I asked them to pick a disease state that they have had personal and/or familial experience with for the application process. Within that real-life context, the student becomes more interested and able to work through application of theory or research. This approach also circles back to Bergmann and Sams' (2014) statement that "flipped learning, at its core, is individualized learning" (p. 7). Even though there are many ways to create a student-centered learning environment, flipped learning provides a unique opportunity to change the focus of your classroom from the educator to the learner. We already know the material, so why should our classroom be focused on us as the educators? We need to work to focus our classroom on our learner who is in need of knowledge development instead.

What If My Students Don't Want the Flipped Classroom?

It is possible that even with a solid plan to prepare students for the flipped classroom, there may be some existing resistance from students as they begin to understand the work and dedication involved. Even the highest motivation or sense of urgency to learn the material has the potential to be overshadowed by the realization of the work that is associated with success in learning it. Talbert (2015) speaks of this student resistance to the flipped classroom and proposes that many of the students rebelling are doing so because they want professors to lecture to them and tell them exactly how to earn a "good grade." His article about student resistance to flipped learning makes three very important points about the most typical of student complaints.

Talbert's (2015) first point is that many students feel that the flipped classroom does not provide them the direct instruction that they would traditionally get from a lecture. There is no lack of lecture in the flipped classroom. The lecture is simply watched at home on the video rather than watched live in the classroom. There is in fact a great deal of direct instruction lecture going on in a flipped classroom, but it is not taking place when the students and instructor are together during assigned class time. The additional benefit of having lecture material recorded lies in the ability to watch the lecture over and over again if desired. Students can also pause or rewind the lecture if they missed an important point. In many ways, the flipped classroom recorded lecture is more available and at the students' fingertips than ever before. Students have mentioned that they often go back and listen to each lecture again when they are studying for an exam. Direct instruction that the students in Talbert's study thought was missing, is actually much more available to them in the active learning flipped classroom. While teaching groups of students or individuals during the in-class activities, nurse educators are able to address individual misconceptions and learning needs of each student. When viewed from this lens, the flipped classroom augments direct instruction of each student in the classroom.

Talbert's (2015) second point is that students want lecture because they feel it is the only way for them to earn a top grade in the class. Students (especially nursing students) want to get an "A" in the class and that is an honorable goal. But does this really reflect the amount of learning that has occurred by each student? Does the "A" in the coursework necessarily translate into the best nurses? Is the "A" our students' definition of success? Talbert believes that we can help students define their success in the course in ways other than the course or exam grade. For this reason, he encourages fellow educators to use more to assess student learning than quizzing and testing. If the only assessments used in the course are quizzes and tests, the students will be focused on quizzes and tests as their measure of success in the course. Perhaps this is an area where partnering with the students to arrive at a collaborative set of evaluation ideas would be beneficial to reframing the way nursing students define success in a course. Even if the students' contribution for objectives and subsequent evaluation is only for the 20% genius time that Bergmann and Sams' (2014) have discussed, it might go a long way in terms of allowing them to express their passions and motivation to learn.

One might add to Talbert's suggestion that nurse educators could be asking the students what success looks from their point of view. If they respond that it is an "A" in the course, perhaps we could suggest that they already get an "A" and therefore begin the course successful. What they accomplish within the course will determine whether they keep the "A" or lose it. Could taking this goal off of the table free up that perpetual competition of nursing students who believe that a certain grade is the only way they can define success in a course? Could it allow more room to make learning and retaining information part of their definition of success? Better yet, their success marker could be becoming the best nurses they possibly can be. Perhaps changing the target of what academic success actually means has the potential to motivate students in a new and more rounded way.

Talbert's (2015) third point feeds directly into the discussion of this chapter. He believes that the main reason students are resistant to the flipped classroom boils down to their uncertainty with the method. It changes the rules of the game that they have become very astute at playing. They have acclimated themselves to the lecture altitude. Changing the lecture model into the flipped classroom "violates their expectations and introduces a lot of uncertainty—and conflict can be a coping mechanism" (2015, p. 17). Talbert suggests that if students are being rebellious to the flipped classroom, they are exactly where you want them to be. When they are forced to break out of their educational comfort zone, they are primed to learn about learning and the value of learning over the value of a grade. Helping students to ease into the process slowly using a change theory model such as Kotter's (2015) has the potential to help with student uncertainty and mistrust with the use of the flipped classroom.

Step 2: Build a Guiding Coalition

Kotter (2015) describes Step 2, *Build a Guiding Coalition,* of the process for leading change as "assembling a group with the power and energy to lead and support a collaborative change effort."

The nurse educator will be the main change agent in the flipped classroom scenario, but may be working with other educators in the same course. If this is the case, all can work together to form the flipped classroom piece by piece. Kotter's second step of change can also be accomplished by building a network of educators from which to share ideas, successes, and common frustrations. Working with other educators toward the goal of successful flipping can bring about a great deal of support and creative effort in the process of implementing the flipped classroom.

An important part of building a coalition may be talking with your director or dean about the idea to flip your classroom. With the documented amount of student resistance and strong reliance on student evaluations for faculty annual review, it would be a good idea to have a conversation about your ideas with the person in charge. The conversation might include any known physical or personnel needs that you would like to request these leadership. The good software packages can be expensive, but many institutions carry a licensure that nurse educators can take advantage of. Although not all nursing programs have the resources, asking for a graduate assistant and a physical space for students to conduct their group work are reasonable requests. The lack of physical space can be a big challenge when flipping the classroom. These specific needs for flipping the classroom may be those that can be envisioned ahead of time and discussed with leadership accordingly.

Step 3: Form a Strategic Vision and Initiatives and Step 4: Enlist Volunteer Army

Step 3, *Form a Strategic Vision and Initiatives,* is described by Kotter (2015) as "shape a vision to help steer the change effort and develop strategic initiatives to achieve that vision." Step 4, *Enlist Volunteer Army*, is described as very similar, "raise a large force of people who are ready, willing and urgent to drive change" (2015).

For nursing educators, this powerful group and volunteer army equates to nursing student groups. For both faculty and students, Steps 3 and 4 can involve the partnering process discussed earlier. Prensky (2010) recommends that in partnering, the teacher asks great questions and the students search for the answers or the students are given a topic or subject and ask the questions that they then will answer. Prensky's discussion of the common way textbooks are developed with chapter questions at the back of each chapter rather than at the front is interesting. This format does not allow for the student to engage their brain and begin to think through problems and answers on their own ahead of time or during their reading. Instead, it provides all the answers up front, and then questions the student about their knowledge of the given answers within the chapter at the end. Prensky has a point that the way textbooks are formatted does have the potential to stunt creative and critical thinking. Perhaps we can use the textbooks in a more thought-provoking rather than thought-giving manner. In our world of evidence-based practice, the textbook can be used as one source along with articles and current research on the topic. Many nurse educators are most likely already using this approach.

A Poor Example of Partnering With Students

To begin the discussion about partnering with students, I would first like to share with you an example of when partnering with students was not considered. It happens to be the first time I flipped the classroom as well. My colleague and I did have some forethought about preparing the students who were in unchanging cohorts throughout the program. The cohort model allowed us to visit the students in December prior to the spring semester start. We took about 15 minutes to explain the flipped classroom to them, how it would be different, and how we thought it would improve our ability to teach them about the clinical world that they would encounter during the clinical portion of the course. We had few questions from the group, and several vertical bobbing student heads that we took as a sign of approval and interest. Although this was a good place to start preparing our students, we soon found that we fell far short of ensuring their understanding and buy-in of our use of the flipped classroom method.

We did take a bit of time the first day of class to re-introduce the method to the students. To our surprise, the majority of them did not remember our discussion in December. They said that they remember us coming to talk to them, but didn't recall exactly what we had told them. In hindsight, the timing of our introduction to the method was not well planned. While we were trying to tell them about the flipped classroom, the students had been given the course evaluations for the current semester, so some of them were busy with this task. They had also just finished a big review for their upcoming final the next week. It was easy to see how they might have been preoccupied with other thoughts and filled with attention-stealing stress. Some were very honest with us, telling us that when we talked with them they were not really concerned about the up and coming semester. Instead, they were trying to survive the current semester with a passing grade.

After a reintroduction of the method, we did have a few questions from students focused mostly around how their readings would be cut back in order to allow for time to watch any posted videos. We shared that the readings would not change. This information upset the students because they saw videos as additional homework time that they would not have if lecture was the main form of instruction. Their immediate concern was not about their learning, but about how much work the course was going to be for them outside of the classroom. Most of the students have some sort of family or other social commitments and work full-time or almost full-time while attempting to complete graduate studies. It is completely understandable that students would have concerns about more required work outside the classroom. We again explained how we believed that the flipped classroom could really help them address more realistic clinical questions and be more prepared for the type of testing we would be doing later on in the course. The students agreed mostly because we did not give them any other option or allow them to partner to help us make the class more of what they wanted in their learning experience.

Similar nursing student resistance to the flipped classroom can be found in the existing literature. Missildine, Fountain, Summers, and Gosselin (2013) found in their study on flipping an adult health BSN course, that students had lower satisfaction scores for anything but lecture. The authors stated that with their use of lecture capture and small group work with students, they were able to model and engage their students in development of clinical reasoning, reflection, application of up-to-date research, and expansion of their clinical imagination. Their study goes a long way in proving a point that more innovative methods in the classroom can result in improved learning but not necessarily improved student satisfaction. It is also important to remember Benner and colleagues' statement that what students like in a class may not be what they need (Benner, Sutphen, Leonard, & Day, 2010).

Similar to a study by Schwartz (2014), our students did get used to the flipped classroom as the semester progressed. At first our students were quite upset that lecture was not being delivered because in literally every class they had taken to that point. Herein lies the challenge of attempting any new method of teaching and learning that requires more active student-focused learning instead of passive learning by lecture. Our students did interpret the flipped model as requiring more work from them than a traditional lecture format, and they were correct. The flipped classroom moves the work in the classroom to student-centered from educator-centered. As this shift occurs, the students will have to be more active and self-directed in their learning process. Coupled with the discomfort that accompanies any change, the flipped classroom may bring distress to the students. It would be helpful to have more research focused on student satisfaction associated with the flipped learning model. But our students also admitted at the end of the course that they had experienced a deeper, more intense learning during the course than they had in previous courses. For this they were appreciative. One student reported that she felt very well prepared to take care of pediatric and obstetric patients in the clinical setting due to the heavy use of case studies and real-life scenarios in the flipped classroom. She also mentioned that she felt more grounded in understanding what important questions to ask, and how to find answers to those questions on her own. These are important clinical skills for a beginning FNP. I consider this very valuable and positive feedback that I had not received when the course was straight lecture.

A Better Example of Partnering

Now I would like to take some time to share a very positive partnering experience with my students. It also provides an example of how we can use partnering to enlist our students in the change process involved with flipped learning.

A couple of years back I was assigned one of our undergraduate nursing core courses as a new part of my teaching assignment about a month prior to the semester beginning due to some faculty leaving unexpectedly. I was immediately resistant because I had heard from others teaching this same course that the students *always* hated the content, so whoever taught the course was pretty much guaranteed to get a poor set of student evaluations. One faculty member who taught the course regularly reported in her annual evaluation that she was not able to get high student evaluation scores because the content was just not "sexy" enough. I actually laughed out loud, but at the same time did understand what she was talking about, having taught this type of course in the past. The main concepts in the course were evidence-based practice, the research process, ethics, cultural context of care, and patient teaching.

Needless to say, I was pretty unprepared to teach this core course to our second-semester junior students. Other than my current FNP practice with various cultural groups, my past teaching experience, and ability to do research, I felt fairly ill equipped. I found out that this was actually a blessing for me as the instructor. I reviewed the existing syllabus and began to think about how I would deliver this supposedly doomed content to the students. I had some ideas, but wasn't sure how I might be able to really engage the students when teaching this content. It was during this contemplation I realized that to be able to interest them, I needed to know more about them. The students were second-degree students, all coming to the nursing bachelors program with a previous degree. How could I use their past experiences and expertise to make this course content more applicable and interesting to them while showing them how use of this content was a valuable part of their nursing practice?

The first day of class we went through everyone introducing themselves to me. You may have done this in your own classes to get a better idea of who you are teaching. As the students introduced themselves one by one, I began to realize the wealth of experience in the classroom. These students were second-degree students, all having some sort of professional life or degree prior to beginning their nursing education. I also became keenly aware that this group of students had been together for 4 semesters prior to this course, and had formed a culture to which I was an outsider. I am an ethnographer and recognized that I needed to form some sort of coalition with this group to become a part of their culture. This was my serendipitous segue into Kotter's Steps 2 and 4.

After the introductions, I stood in front of the class as planned and went through the syllabus page by page. After this, I changed the focus and put the ball in their court. I began to have a conversation with the students about their expectations for the course. I asked them what they wanted to do in the course. How did they want to meet the learning objectives that had been set by the undergraduate curriculum committee? At first they thought I was joking. I reassured them and said that as long as we met the objectives of the course, we could do it the way we wanted to. I also had to keep some of the assignments for the course the same in order to be similar to the other section of the course—this was dictated to me by the assistant director, so it was not negotiable. The ideas that these students brought forth were incredible. It was the first time that I began to understand what kind of people I was teaching: very capable, full of great ideas, wanting to learn but in their own way, and full of energy once they had a chance to be a part of their learning process. I was immediately energized about this course and the material. What a switch in my attitude and I think it was a switch for the students' attitudes as well.

I think part of this success story had to do with my comfort level to be "real" with my students. I told them that this course had a notorious bad rap among our faculty. I shared with them that I was concerned about their engagement with the material because it was touted as "not sexy enough" to keep student attention. They thought this was actually pretty funny, but had also heard from other student groups that the course was boring and barely tolerable. As a result, I had them describe to me what was considered "sexy" content in their professional nursing student opinion. As each student came forth with their own idea of what would constitute "sexy" content, I responded showing them how the concepts within the course would help them to employ that specific, more "sexy," content. Remember, I had not planned this—it just happened in a most wonderful way.

After this conversation, I talked to them about how a supermodel might prepare for the runway walk or how an actress might prepare for a specific scene. They responded that there must be an entourage of people who do the hair, makeup, dress the actress or model, and put her in the best possible light to appear the way she does in the film or on stage. I used this as an analogy for our course. The course concepts, although not "sexy" on their own, would be the entourage that would create the "sexy" appearance of the more sensational nursing actions. In this way, I was able to make the content applicable and more interesting to them on the first day—all by just being real and asking for their input. I had to ask them about their ideas and their opinions in order to match their ideas with those about the applicability of the content for the semester. I think this is a good example of partnering at its best.

The comment and following discussion about "sexy" nursing content became our own little inside joke throughout the course. At the end of the course, about 80% of the student evaluations had a similar write in comment, "Karen made this the sexiest nursing course I have ever taken!" Needless to say, I had to explain this to my director! I had excellent student evaluations, and more positive comments than ever before, all because I partnered with my students and engaged them in their learning process. I also approached my students as colleagues in the teaching/learning process rather than exercising the unspoken power that can benefit a higher education instructor.

When I allowed them to have some sort of power in their learning process, it changed the whole atmosphere for the course.

I didn't find Prensky's (2010) work about teaching digital natives and partnering with students until after I had begun flipping the classroom. Much of what he recommended aligns with the example of partnering provided above. In his text, Prensky suggested that letting the students do what they do best includes allowing them to find and follow their passion and practicing material with games and activities. His set of suggestions for instructors using the partnering framework includes creating and asking the right questions and giving students guidance. Nurse educators are also responsible for creating rigor and ensuring quality, as you might expect. When working with students within this type of framework, there is a lot of room for negotiation of learning approach with student groups. Negotiation with students on how to meet the learning objectives has the potential to get them more involved with the process of learning. As Prensky states, "partnering is the very opposite of teaching by telling... Rather than lecture or even explain, the teacher needs only give students, in a variety of ways, questions to be answered..." (2010, p. 13).

Step 5: Enable Action by Removing Barriers

Step 5, *Enable Action by Removing Barriers,* is "to remove obstacles to change, change systems or structures that pose threats to the achievement of the vision" (Kotter, 2015).

It is no secret that there are some barriers to nursing students' acceptance of the flipped classroom. Helping students understand how the flipped classroom can help their learning in your course can go a long way in removing their resistance. Using the information provided by Talbert (2015), we can think ahead and address each of the most common concerns students have about flipping the classroom.

Lack of knowledge about the flipped classroom is likely among nursing student populations. As Talbert (2015) discussed, students are likely to have a fair amount of uncertainty and mistrust with the method as a result. Educating them on what the flipped classroom is and does can help to decrease this anxiety. Sharing a short video about the flipped classroom with students may provide a helpful opening dialogue to more education about the flipped classroom. There are several short and very informative videos on the Internet that can be of help. The videos that have been created by Bergmann and Sams (2014) are the most useful. They are very well done, entertaining, and come from the pioneers of the method. It is helpful that I teach in Colorado, because Bergmann and Sams are from the same state. Students like that such innovation came from within their own state and share a bit of pride associated with being in the pioneering state.

Also highly recommend are the videos available on The Flipped Learning Network (2015). They are informative, very well done, and created by Bergmann and Sams (2014) as well. I particularly like the video titled "A Video Introduction to the Foundations of Flipped Learning" (2015), but there are several available that are terrific to view for students and faculty. These videos can be found under the "Resources" tab on the main webpage.

After showing students a video, begin a conversation with your students about their thoughts and concerns with the flipped classroom. One idea to get this conversation going, it to provide each student with a sheet of paper that has 3 main fill-in sections:

1. *What do you like about the idea of the flipped classroom?*
2. *Why do you not like the idea of the flipped classroom? Be specific.*
3. *How would you define "success" in this course?*

Have the students take about 5 minutes to write down their thoughts and ask them not to put their names on the sheets of paper. Have one student volunteer go to the board (or do it yourself) to make a list of positives and concerns. Be careful not to use the word *negatives* in this process. Keep it positive! Begin by reading each of the positive thoughts from students and tally up the ones that are repetitive. Move to what the students are concerned about and discuss this list as well. At this time, attempt to reassure students about their concerns and how you will be sure to address them along the way. Lastly, have a discussion about how students define success in your course.

The two most common things students are concerned about are that they will not know what is going to be on a test and that they will have too much work to do at home preparing for class. Reassure them with the fact that you have preset learning objectives and will be focused on those learning objectives for each unit of the course. This is and always has been how they will know what is on the test and is not different with the flipped classroom. Of course, they might not necessarily like this explanation, but it does address their concern about testing, which is a big concern among students. You may also discuss how you will be able to use their time in class together to better prepare them for not only their tests but for the interactions they are likely to encounter in their clinical settings. At all costs, keep things positive! Don't allow any negativity to enter the conversation. Always address a negative thought or comment with a positive one about the flipped classroom. Positivity is infectious, and if you are positive, your students are likely to become more positive as well.

If you will recall, another of the most common complaints of students about the flipped classroom is rooted in their perception that they are not receiving direct instruction. If they are not experiencing that lecture in the classroom, they are more cautious and resistant of the method (Talbert, 2015). It is, after all, a major change in their expectations of you as their faculty member if they use their previous educational experience as a measuring stick. During the conversation about concerns this may come up. First of all, remind them that they will still be having lecture. The lecture will now be on a lecture video that they can watch over and over, pause, and rewind. Most students like this idea of having the lecture more available to them. Talk to your students about your ability to address their learning needs one on one with the class time rather than using group instruction with limited or no individual instruction time during a lecture. You have a very good argument that the flipped classroom allows you to do your job of teaching them much more effectively. You can be certain to reach each and every student and conduct real-time assessment of their understanding of the material. You can also allow them to have some flexibility in the ways they want to learn and meet the learning objectives. Even if they are not convinced on that first day, they will be armed with some good information and ideas about what they are about to do in the flipped classroom that will be different than their past lecture-based courses.

Dr. Jerry Overmyer of the Flipped Learning Network and lead of the Flipped Learning Academy at the University of Northern Colorado (UNC) has an excellent idea of how to show students firsthand how the flipped classroom will be helpful for their learning: *The Origami Frog Project* (see **Figure 5-2**).

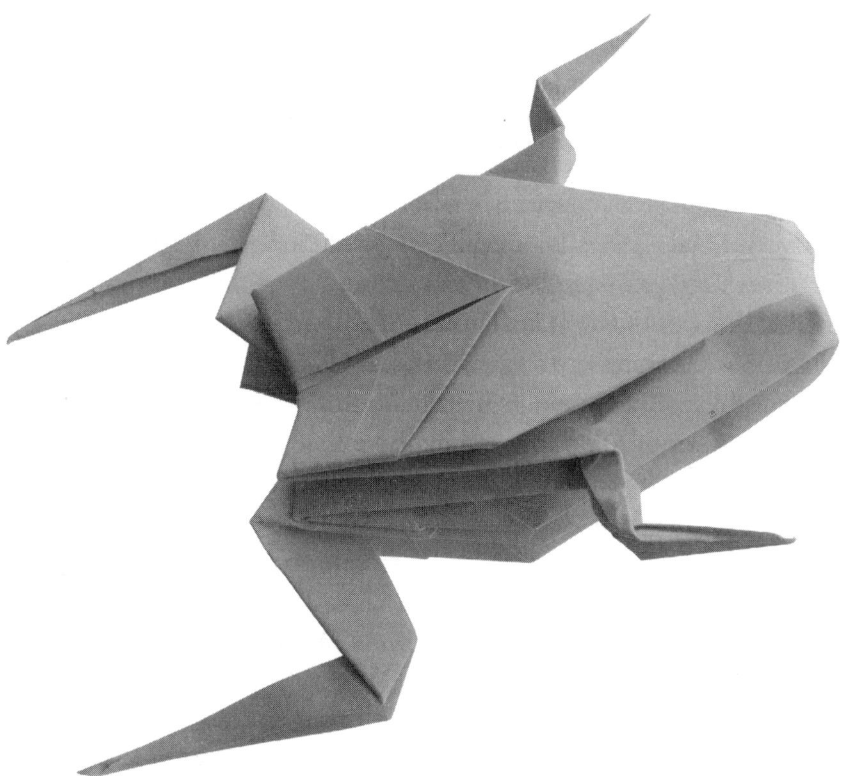

Figure 5-2 Origami Frog Project.

About a week prior to the class starting, use the e-mail list provided for your students to send out a video on how to make an origami frog out of a piece of plain copy paper to about half of the students on your list. Instruct them in the e-mail to complete their origami frog prior to coming to class. Have them bring their completed frog to class the first day for the first assignment of the course. The remaining half of the students will receive no e-mail about the assignment. Try to choose a video that does the frog quickly, not giving much time at all to get the concept. The video does not have to be a origami frog, you could choose a more complex fold such as a butterfly or star to turn up the complexity a bit. The first day of class, provide each student a piece of plain paper and tell them that they must construct the origami frog while you play the same video you sent to the students ahead of time. Those who have done this at home will already have their frog and will be ready to go. Those who do not have their frog made will need to watch the video in real time and create the frog on the spot.

During our faculty Flipped Learning Academy at UNC, Jerry had us complete this very task. I will tell you that we all got lost trying to watch that video of how to make the frog in real time. We kept saying, "Go back, I missed something." But he would not stop the video. As a result, none of us had a correctly made frog at the end of the video and we were all frustrated and lost. Here is a perfect example of how having the video ahead of time and being able to use it at an individualized pace of understanding can be valuable to learning any material. I think that this is an absolutely brilliant idea, and one that can show the students that flipped learning is a positive thing for them to be a part of.

Along the same lines as the idea of the origami frog, a short video lecture could be sent to the other half of the students prior to the first day of class. Of course, the origami frog students will not receive this e-mail. The video should be directly related to a couple of learning objectives about the content for the course. For example, an undergraduate physical assessment course video could cover the difference between subjective and objective data within the patient's health history and history of present illness. During the class, have the students complete a written assignment or even a verbal assignment as a group to differentiate subjective from objective information. This might be a good place to use the automated response system with quiz-type material for your class. The students who have watched the short video prior to the class will be ahead of the game and able to answer the questions or complete a written or group assignment with much more ease than those who did not have access to the video. Using these types of real-time and hands-on strategies to show the students the benefit of the flipped classroom can be extremely helpful.

Step 6: Generate Short-Term Wins

Step 6, *Generate Short-Term Wins,* is defined as "to consistently produce, track, evaluate, and celebrate volumes of small and large accomplishments – and correlate them to results" (Kotter, 2015).

Using these examples of how to orient students to the flipped classroom can begin a generation of short-term wins. This particular step of Kotter's preparation for change may be focused on how the students met the learning objectives within the new pedagogy. Sharing with the students the short- and long-term wins in terms of knowledge acquisition is one of the best ways to celebrate. You may want to negotiate ahead of time what these short-term wins will be for you and your students. Partner with them to choose a "reward" for completing the first flipped classroom, or negotiate a short-term "win" for them after the first exam is passed by all. Short-term wins can be as simple as having class outside for the day, weather permitting, or allowing the students to brainstorm their own ideas of what they would choose as a celebration.

The other part of Kotter's Step 6 relates more to the role of faculty member. As faculty members embarking on a change in pedagogy, we are in an ideal position to gather data on the process and outcomes, and publish that data for our nursing peers. Consider conducting some research on your flipped classroom. I understand that this is a repetitive suggestion, but an important one. Perhaps partnering with another researcher in your area or institution that has some research experience would be an option if faculty members do not yet possess a research degree themselves. It would also be a fantastic research focus for any students desiring to conduct educational research. Collaboration on these types of scholarship of teaching and learning projects can be quite informative to the nursing education community at large.

Step 7: Sustain Acceleration

Step 7, *Sustain Acceleration,* is to "use increasing credibility to change systems, structures and policies that don't align with the vision; hire, promote and develop employees who can implement the vision; reinvigorate the process with the new projects, themes and volunteers" (Kotter, 2015).

Although the description of Step 7 by Kotter is directed primarily toward the business or corporate world, it can be translated to the flipped classroom process of change. Once the initial flipped classroom has become a success, Kotter would suggest that we move forward and continue to flip more and more classes. Changing structures and policies that don't align with the flipped classroom can be as simple as altering the learning objectives with help or blessing of the nursing curriculum committee.

Changing the policies for the flipped classroom can also be completed by altering the syllabus to include flipped learning objectives and learning outcome assessments. The syllabus should reflect use of the flipped classroom. If you are comfortable with the idea of allowing students to have some flexibility to follow their individual passions, be certain to include this type of agreement into the syllabus. As previously mentioned, the ideas can originate from the students, but the rigor and guidance need to come from the faculty teaching the course. Provide some structure for assignments, but consider allowing students to choose the subject matter. The idea of a selective menu of assignments to complete the learning objectives is a popular idea among students. Some students may prefer writing a paper about the topic while others may be more interested in developing a class presentation. Some students may prefer to work alone while others like to work within a group. Allowing for students to make these choices can bolster their creativity and ability to work on something that they are passionate about. I would caution that these types of assignments must be clearly outlined for students to avoid any conflicts regarding the end outcome. Well-written rubrics provide a grading expectation for students and are highly encouraged.

Step 8: Institute Change

Step 8, *Institute Change*, is to "articulate the connections between the new behaviors and organizational success, and develop the means to ensure leadership development and succession" (Kotter, 2015).

As you work through the process of flipping the classroom, think about creating a reflective journal. Having students write about their experience in the class may also be of benefit. Reflective journaling can be a mirror of the process, thoughts along the way, and reflections on how to improve the process. The reflective journal does not need to be expansive by any means. Saving the last 5 to 10 minutes of class for journaling of thoughts about the process and what each has learned in the class can be very productive.

As introduced by Schon (1983), reflective practice is described as a process in which a professional attempts a new approach, reflects upon that approach in action, alters the approach as necessary (sometimes in real time), and reflects on the process after completion. Becoming a reflective practitioner and educator can foster an attitude of perpetual analysis and the idea of refining our approach as we are acting. Reflective journaling is a process that provides a record of this reflective process. Reflective journaling can foster thinking in action, and development of a self-analysis of either process or learning. Schuessler, Wilder, and Byrd (2012) found that reflective journaling helped their students to progressively develop critical thinking and self-reflection skills, and develop a sense of cultural humility.

The one thing that may be missing in Kotter's 8-step process is such a reflective element and the idea of continuous quality improvement. Keeping a reflective journal can assist with Kotter's suggestion to find connections between the flipped classroom and associated successes. Conversely, it can reveal areas that were not as successful and are in need of revision. The journal provides a written mirror of the process and self-feedback along the way for both instructor and student. Using this feedback and reflection can become part of the evaluation process of the Intentional Instruction Model that will be covered in an upcoming chapter.

When faculty share their abilities, experiences, and ideas with other nurse educators, the second part of Kotter's step 8 can be accomplished. Providing leadership and mentorship to other nurse educators that desire to flip their courses leads to more use of the method. More use of the method will hopefully lead to more solid research about using the flipped classroom in the field of nursing education. Once you have flipped your classroom and feel confident in your abilities, share that with others and help them to be successful as well.

Conclusion

Preparing students for the flipped classroom takes time and a carefully constructed plan. Taking the time to anticipate student fears and concerns and addressing them up front can be a great prevention strategy in terms of student resistance to using the method. Helping students to understand that you are for them and not against them is an important step in this process as well. The highly competitive nature of even getting accepted into a nursing program may cause our students to think of nursing faculty as some kind of enemy when the exact opposite is true. Many nursing programs admit students on the basis of grade point average. Although this is an accepted method of admission, it can set up a strong spirit of competition among pre-nursing students. Once they are accepted into a nursing program, they tend to carry this competitive spirit and anxiety with them.

Many first semester nursing students have shared with me that there is a general perception among pre-clinical nursing majors that pre-requisite courses for nursing programs exist to "weed out the herd" of nursing program applicants. Due to this strong competitive atmosphere, nursing students tend to be mistrusting and think of faculty as globally attempting to separate the strong students from the weak in some manner. As faculty we can't help but understand and empathize with our students as they worry about being the next person voted off the island. As nursing faculty, we can create an atmosphere of caring, mentoring, and partnership with our soon-to-be colleagues to help dispel this type of misperception. Using the flipped classroom can help nursing faculty to gain a better appreciation of who each student is, what they hold as their passion, and how we can assist in their individual learning from day to day.

References

Benner, P., Sutphen, M., Leonard, V., & Day, L. (2010). *Education nurses: A call for radical transformation.* Stanford, CA: The Carnegie Foundation for the Advancement of Teaching.

Bergmann, J., & Sams, A. (2014). *Flipped learning: Gateway to student engagement.* Eugene, OR: International Society for Technology in Education.

Hendry, G. D, Hyde, S. J., & Davy, P. (2005). Independent study groups. *Medical Education, 39* (7), 672–679.

Kotter, J. (2015). The 8-step process for leading change. Retrieved from http://www.kotterinternational.com/the-8-step-process-for-leading-change/

Missildine K., Fountain R., Summers, L., & Gosselin, K. (2013). Flipping the classroom to improve student performance and satisfaction. *Journal of Nursing Education, 52*(10), 597–599.

Prensky, M. (2010). *Teaching digital natives: Partnering for real learning*. Thousand Oaks, CA: Corwin SAGE.

Schuessler, J. B., Wilder, B., & Byrd, L. W. (2012). Reflective journaling and development of cultural humility in students. *Nursing Education Perspectives, 33*(2), 96–99.

Schwartz, T. A. (2014). Flipping the statistics classroom in nursing education. *Journal of Nursing Education, 53*(4), 199–206.

Schon, D. A. (1983). The reflective practitioner: *How professionals think in action*. New York, NY: Basic Books.

Swellar, J., van Merrienboer, J., & Paas, F. (1998). Cognitive architecture and instructional design. *Educational Psychology Review, 10*(3), 251–296.

Talbert, R. (2015, January). Flipped learning skepticism: Do students want to have lectures? *The Chronicle of Higher Education*, 15–17.

The Flipped Learning Network. (2015). Retrieved from http://flippedlearning.org/site/default.aspx?PageID=1

CHAPTER 6

Off-Load Content—What Will Students Do Prior to Class?

Introduction

As described in the Intentional Instruction Model (**Figure 6-1**), off-load content is any material that students will be accessing and completing prior to coming to the face-to-face or live class to interact with the instructor. The content chosen as off-load should flow directly from the objectives for the class and be a building block for the in-class learning strategies. One of the most unique features of the flipped classroom that makes it different than other forms of active learning is the movement of the group learning portion of a course, such as lecture, into the off-load material for students to access prior to the face-to-face class time. Use of video capture software has allowed ease of delivery of lecture-based learning into off-load material. However, video lectures are not the only off-load material available for use within the flipped classroom. Off-load materials can include other assignments and individual learning experiences, all of which will be discussed within this chapter.

General Guidelines for Development of Off-Load Material

When creating a solid plan for flipping the classroom, an understanding of how all the different parts of the Intentional Instruction

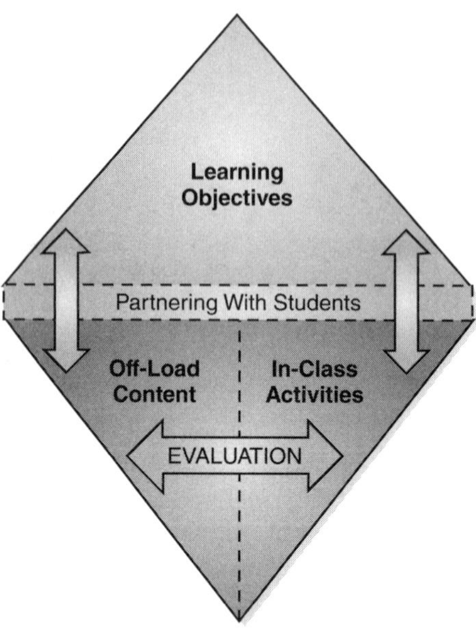

Figure 6-1 The Intentional Instruction Model for Flipped Learning.

Model for Flipped Learning are connected is essential. As previously mentioned, the objectives should provide the roadmap for the flipped classroom experience. As discussed in a previous chapter, part of faculty preparation for the flipped classroom involves taking time to separate the learning objectives that are lower ordered and directed toward student self-learning from those that are higher ordered and require more critical thinking and analysis. In the flipped classroom, the lower-ordered learning objectives are perfect for development of the off-load materials. The flipped classroom works best when the objectives that require higher-ordered critical thinking skills from the students are saved for the in-class portion of learning time. This structure allows faculty to help students through more complex learning.

When Bloom's Taxonomy terms are used to assist in the planning of off-load materials, defining, describing, explaining, repeating, recognizing, or identifying information are words used to describe lower-level objectives. It is interesting that teaching strategies such

Suggested Instructional Strategies for Use with Each Level of Bloom's Taxonomy

lecture
visuals
video
audio
examples
illustrations
analogies

KNOWLEDGE

define
repeat
record
list

questions
discussion
review
test
assessment
reports
learner
presentations
writing

COMPREHENSION

translate
restate
discuss
describe
recognize
explain
express
identify

exercises
practice
demonstrations
projects
sketches
simulations
role play
microteach

APPLICATION

interpret
apply
employ
use
demonstrate
dramatize
practice
illustrate
operate
schedule
shop
sketch

problems
exercises
case studies
critical incidents
discussion
questions
test

ANALYSIS

distinguish
analyze
differentiate
appraise
calculate
experiment
test
compare
contrast
criticize
diagram
inspect
debate
inventory
question
relate

projects
problems
case studies
creative exercises
develop plans
constructs
simulations

SYNTHESIS

compose
plan
propose
design
formulate
arrange
collect
construct
create
set up
organize
manage
prepare

case studies
projects
exercises
critiques
simulations
appraisals

EVALUATION

judge
appraise
evaluate
rate
compare
value
revise
score
select
choose
assess
estimate
measure

Figure 6-2 Bloom's Taxonomy Terms.
Natural Resources Conservation Service

as lecture, videos, tests, writing, and presentations are associated with these lower-level objectives and associated taxonomy. **Figure 6-2** provides a very nice list of teaching strategies to choose from as one plans the off-load portion of the flipped classroom.

As the student is asked to begin applying, analyzing, and/or synthesizing the information, it is most beneficial to have the nursing instructor there to help maneuver the higher-ordered, more-complicated objectives. Much of the in-class time of my flipped classroom is focused on the use of real-life case studies of patients and families seen in the clinical setting. Note from the Bloom's Taxonomy (Figure 6-2), use of a case study requires that a student be able to apply, analyze, and synthesize the information. It also suggests that a student must form questions for the instructor and fellow students about the topic to stimulate discussion and deeper understanding. When students get

Consider This...

If you are only using lecture to teach your students, you are teaching them at the lowest level of Bloom's Taxonomy.

to the point of asking complex questions about patient care based on what will be seen in the clinical setting, they move into the realm of experiential learning. Although they are not in the clinical setting during the in-class portion of the flipped classroom, such low-fidelity simulation moves students onto the first step of the experiential learning ladder. According to Cognitive Load Theory (Swellar, van Merrienboer, & Paas, 1998) and Benner's Novice to Expert Theory (2001), students gain more knowledge and expertise as they are exposed to experiences that put them into real-life scenarios. When students work to critically think through clinical scenarios, it takes them closer to the clinical environment and hones their clinical decision skills. Each nursing action a student performs in the clinical setting is first prompted by critical thinking and reasoning. Providing this type of clinical simulation during in-class case studies in a safe environment to exercise the skills of critical thinking and reasoning can be a powerful learning tool for nursing students.

Although this chapter is focused on discussing the planning and ideas for off-load content separately, it is important to remember that off-load is only one piece of the flipping puzzle that must match with all other pieces for the best teaching/learning to occur. In the most effective flipped classroom, the class objectives drive the off-load assignments and in-class learning strategies. The in-class activities build upon what was assigned in the off-load materials. The evaluation provides a picture of whether or not the learning objectives were met.

Use Off-Load Appropriately

One important point about off-load material use within the model of the flipped classroom must be understood. Use of off-load materials and assignments to increase the amount of material for students or address additional objectives due to lack of class time is a common mistake of some flipping instructors. The main goal of the flipped classroom is not to increase the workload of the students or cover more objectives. Instead, the goal of off-load materials should be to prepare students to learn in a stepwise fashion. The off-load materials and assignments specifically use the lower-ordered learning objectives that can be mastered by individuals prior to in-class time.

I want to share with you a conversation I had with another nursing instructor at a conference where I was presenting on the flipped classroom. She was very excited about use of video lecture, and came up to discuss the capabilities after the presentation. I remember her comment about using the lecture capture to put additional material online for students that she didn't have time for in the classroom. After further discussion I found that she was not planning on using lecture capture videos for the flipped classroom at all. Instead, she was planning to use lecture capture to increase the amount of lecture she was able to expose her students to. *This is not the purpose of video lectures in the context of the flipped classroom.* With these types of misconceptions, it is easy to see why some students and faculty might be resistant to the flipped classroom as an effective pedagogy.

No doubt there is a temptation to use the off-load material to assist nurse educators with the impossible task of covering everything within a bloated nursing curriculum. But the real goal of the pedagogy is to use the face-to-face time faculty have with students to assist them with application of the material. Nurse educators want the time to engage students in the classroom and teach them on a deeper level or allow them to develop a deeper understanding. Moving the large-group teaching strategy of lecture to the individual student via video frees up that face-to-face class time for application and analysis, higher-ordered thinking, and practical application while the faculty are there to assist.

Description of Off-Load Materials for Use With the Flipped Classroom

Video Lectures

Many educators choose to put lecture on videos, which they then assign as off-load content. There are many software programs available for the purpose of recording lectures. Most resources refer to the software as "screen capture software." This term is a generic description of how the software records all movements on the screen during the video. The sound is also recorded and embedded within the video recording. One could spend quite a bit of time finding the screen capture software that works best for them. Like many other computer-based programs, there are features that you may prefer in one program over those in another. Many of the screen capture programs do allow a free trial period for one to access and use the program prior to purchasing. There are some screen capture programs that are free. These programs are limited in their ability in terms of editing and capacity of recording time and storage. They are also typically a shorter, free version of the program that is available for purchase.

When attempting to find the best screen capture software for yourself, a good place to start is the Information Technology (IT) department or teaching and learning support team at your institution. It is possible that there is already an institutional license for one or more of the screen capture software programs that can be taken advantage of. If a technological support team is not available, I would suggest first doing a quick Internet search to see what is available. Providing any specific URL within the pages of this book is risky because URLs have a tendency to change rapidly. However, a good phrase to search would be "screen capture software." After one is armed with some good information, schedule a time to have a conversation with the leadership within the college or school of nursing. Talking to leadership about plans to flip the classroom and needs for support may be extremely fruitful. The leadership may know of other faculty on your campus or even in your department that are using the flipped classroom and could be of help and support, as well.

If one prefers to record videos on a mobile device, there are some apps available that provide screen capture similar to the personal computer options. Many are free, but once again limit the ability to edit, store, and, in most cases, deliver the video once it has been completed. These mobile device apps may be easier to use after proficiency is reached with a personal computer–based program first due to the inability to edit easily. One strategy is to save any set of presentation slides into a PDF and email them to an address that can be opened on the digital device. Once in the mobile device, open the PDF within the screen capture app and it is ready to be turned into a recording. Recordings on mobile devices need to be short because the space to store videos is usually limited.

One caveat about the mobile apps for recording lectures lies in delivery of the video to students. Some of the apps will not allow any video to be transferred outside of that particular app. Due to this feature, each student in your class must have a mobile device and download the app in order to view video. The video lectures recorded with computer-based software can be opened and played on most if not all mobile devices if the students have a mobile device and prefer to use it.

Tips When Recording Your Own Videos

As previously mentioned, students have shared that they like to watch videos that have been recorded by the same faculty that will be teaching them within the face-to-face, live classroom. When recording a lecture for off-load material, there are some important tips to consider. Timing and content to cover in the video are two very important aspects of recording a lecture. The content put into the video will be directly related to how many minutes the video will last. Longer videos create larger video files that are more difficult to upload and share with students. With these thoughts in mind, let's review some key elements of time and content when recording lectures for off-load within the flipped classroom.

Lecture Time ≠ Video Time

Most nursing faculty are accustomed to lecturing during their entire class. Considering that the average nursing course is somewhere around 3 hours per week, this equates to a little less than 3 hours of lecture time total. Off-load video lectures should not be more than 15 to 20 minutes in length. For most nurse educators, this is a math equation that just doesn't add up.

Bergmann and Sams (2012) have suggested that for their K-12 students, lecture videos be less than 15 minutes with a goal of 10 minutes. Most adult nursing students can tolerate a bit more, so a goal of 20 minutes or less per video is best. The caveat here is that this is in no way, shape, or form research-based information. Students in flipped courses have given feedback that in general, 20 minutes is tolerable and 30 minutes or more is close to unbearable. Bergmann and Sams also suggest that one video should only contain one topic. I would agree with this idea in higher education, as well. If a video ends up to be only 10 minutes long, that is a great thing! Don't use this as permission to go back in, edit, and add more content until you get to the 20-minute mark. Quality of what is on the video is far more important than the length. Do not fill the video up with 20 minutes simply because it can be done. Say what needs to be said and send it off.

One lingering question may be "How is it possible to fit 3 hours of lecture into a 15- to 20-minute video?" Well, obviously it is not possible at all. Here is where the expert nurse educator must consider what is in the 3 hours of lecture that is most essential content to deliver to the student in order to address the lower-ordered learning objectives. What is *absolutely necessary* to share with the students about the content? Is there a part of the lecture that is repeating something the students could be reading in an assigned text or article? Is there a part of the lecture that is reviewing material that the students learned in another course? Could there be parts of the lecture, perhaps charts and graphs, that are readily accessible to students in their textbooks or through an article or other online resource?

I will be honest, when I began to ask these same questions about my lectures, I found out some interesting things about what and how I was teaching my students using lecture. Let me give you an example of one of my own lectures and how I was able to break it down to make a video that would prep the students adequately for what I wanted them to do during the face-to-face class period.

One of the classes first flipped was a graduate-level family nurse practitioner course on how to complete an initial pregnancy examination. The original lecture was about 2 hours long and somewhere around 40 slides. After reviewing the lecture in preparation for a shorter video version, it became clear that there was a great deal of repetition of what these students already learned in previous coursework. In several of the presentation slides was a review of female anatomy and physiology, terms associated with pregnancy, and how to complete a female gynecology examination. These students had their physical assessment course the semester prior. Much of what was on this lecture was really re-teaching content that they had already learned and been tested on in the previous course. Some readers might be thinking, "Yes, but students need repetition, it helps them learn." Agreed, but couldn't they do this prior to class, individually, at their own pace, on their own time? Do nurse educators really need to be taking up the precious face-to-face time with students to review content that they've already had in their program of study? One might argue that educators can use the time with students in the classroom much, much more effectively.

As I prepared the slides for the video, I forced myself to delete every slide that contained something the students could read on their own. Instead, the students were referred to their assigned readings. Anything in the lecture that was review material from what the students would have had in previous courses was deleted from the video. In the video it was mentioned that if anyone needed a review of anatomy and physiology or how to complete a GYN examination, they should do that prior to viewing the video. The students were also provided with some review resources and the original slides to form a "review" slide presentation as an additional resource. Later on I did go back to make a recording of the review materials, as well. Students were told that they did not need to watch the review materials unless they thought it was necessary to do so. After paring down the content for the video lecture, the main "take-home" ideas of what was most important to convey to the students was left. The video provided the students with information that could not be found in the readings. For example, the video revealed some clinical pearls personally used in the clinical setting. The video was also focused on adding to the student knowledge base of how to do a GYN exam by comparing it to the initial pregnancy examination. At the end of the video, the assignment for in-class activities was shared. Students were also asked to bring at least one question that they had about the content to class with them for discussion.

It was surprising to find that the end product was a video lecture approximately 15 minutes in length. Everything else the students were directed to read or review by themselves prior to coming to class. Shaving off pieces of any lecture until a skeleton is left is difficult for some instructors. However, doing so does force the nurse educator to focus on that what is really necessary to teach the students about the content using lecture. The rest of what the educator teaches comes during class with application to a case-based scenario or other interactive teaching strategy.

There are times when an educator might find that a 15- or 20-minute lecture video for off-load content is too short. In this case, record 2 separate videos that are shorter in length. Another option is to go ahead and record about 15 or 20 minutes of lecture for off-load and then follow it up with a short burst of lecture at the beginning of the face-to-face class. As each educator becomes more efficient at flipping, they will find that they want to do this less and less. The students prefer getting right down to business testing their knowledge in the application exercises planned for their face-to-face time rather than sitting idly by and listening to lecture. In fact, even these short lectures may become much more of a conversation because students are prompted to ask questions and discuss rather than sit passively in their seats. After everyone has been exposed to the flipped classroom, their tolerance for straight lecture seems to decrease.

Entertaining Videos

When recording screen capture videos, Bergmann and Sams (2012) have suggested that one at least *attempt* to animate their voice to make the video interesting. Even a short video will have students zoning out if it is done with a monotone voice and no inflection during the recording. Bergmann and Sams point out that as educators record more and more videos, they become more relaxed and able to be themselves when recording a video lecture. Agreed, but one may still feel more challenged to be entertaining in front of the computer than when lecturing in front of a group of students. It is surprising to find that talking to a computer is much different than talking to a class during a typical lecture. It is an interesting phenomenon. Using inflection of speech and voice when lecturing in front of a class seems to come more easily than recording the lecture at the computer without a live audience. It is logical that educators have to be somewhat entertaining during a live lecture to keep the attention of the students in the classroom. When alone talking to a computer screen, it is not quite as stimulating. To remedy, we must attempt to think of ourselves as lecturing in the classroom when making the recording in order to make the video as interesting as our live lecture would be.

The lecturing atmosphere is different in a recording versus a live classroom, so it is recommend that some type of bulleted list of what will be said be created prior to sitting down to record. Having a script or bulleted list of important points to discuss for each slide keeps the "dead air" time to a minimum. If there is a long pause while educators stop to think about what they want to say in the video, students could be left with the thought that the audio in the video is no longer working or that the screen froze in some way. Dead air time can also increase the length of any video. It is the goal to start the recording and get through the content within the shortest time possible. Filling the video time with large spaces of "ums" and "I can't think of the word" moments is less than ideal. Having a script also cuts down on any post-recording editing, which can take up a great deal of time, as well.

In addition to creating a script or bulleted list, be certain to not just read what is on the slides to the students. Students can read and do not need to have lecture slides read to them. Of all the soap boxes I have regarding effective instruction, this is probably among the biggest. This is called "PowerPoint karaoke." There is no reason to read slides to students. An educator's job is to use what is on the slides as a bullet point, something to add to or expand upon. For this reason, I find myself using slides for lecture less and less. For the videos, using slides can provide a bulleted list for the video. The slides will help to keep on task and remember what to say during the video. If you decide to make your video using slides, be certain to use the time effectively to expand or add to what is already written. Another approach is to put any bulleted items for the video below the slide in the notes section, and use a picture for the students to look at while discussing. Still another idea, is to make the ideas appear on the slide as they are being discussed. These types of active movements on the screen during a lecture video can assist in maintaining student attention.

Keep It Generic!

When creating lecture videos, think about future classes that will watch the video. Don't put anything specific in the video that would not allow its use again during a subsequent semester. For example, in one of my videos I had remembered that a student in the class had an excellent question, so mentioned it in the video. The video had something like, "Remember that great question about genetics that Sarah asked on Wednesday this week?" Then I used the same video for a subsequent class the following semester, not realizing that little bit of information was still in the video. Needless to say, I had several confused student calls and emails indicating that they didn't know what question Sarah had asked and didn't even know we had a Sarah in the class. We also had class on Thursday that particular semester, so some students were confused as to why class was on Wednesday and wondered if they had missed class. To avoid similar confusion, attempt to keep the discussion in the video only to the topic of the lecture. Doing so will allow use of that same video over and over. When recording lecture videos, also try to not mention time elements (such as winter or summer, or days of the week). In summary, avoid talking in the video about anything that would disallow you from using the very same video in future classes without having to edit.

Using the Webcam

There are some instructors who like to use the webcam to show themselves while recording their lectures. The webcam can be directed only on the lecturing faculty member or can be used with a picture-in-picture feature so that the slides and faculty are showing on the screen together. These types of recording strategies may increase the lecturing video entertainment factor. Others may believe that it serves as more of a distraction and choose not to use the webcam for recordings. One instance in which using the webcam may be appreciated by students would be during an online course. Use of the webcam in the online environment lets the students see their instructor, which might be more personable. My online student feedback is that they appreciate seeing my face during the video. However, if I am going to see my students in class the same week that they watch the video, I don't tend to add myself for a couple of reasons. First of all, adding picture in picture produces added work for me during recording. Secondly, I believe that it provides a point of distraction for students while watching the video. I would rather they focus or concentrate on what I am teaching them on the screen than my talking head. I have also found that it is difficult to get good lighting and synchronous recordings. This is, of course, a personal preference, and you may find that you like the picture in picture and find it to be a very helpful feature in the lecture videos.

Using Humor in Videos

Along the same lines of using voice animation during lecture videos, Bergmann and Sams (2012) recommend that use of a bit of humor in the video is welcomed by students. Using humor in videos sometimes works, but would caution that a purposeful attempt at humor with an adult learning audience can go sour pretty quickly. I do not write humor into any sort of video script, per se, but if something humorous comes about as I record the video, then I don't hesitate to use humor in the video. This humorous opportunity typically comes about as I make a mistake in my video. Instead of editing it out, I usually just poke some fun at myself during the video. The students have commented that they like this type of humor because it shows that I am human. My students have said that they appreciate that there is a personality on the other side of their screen. My students have made the connection that they make their fair share of mistakes, so seeing a bit of humanity in nurse educators can be a comfort to them in a way. I am careful about the use of humor in the videos because I prefer that my videos portray important information about the content rather than a comedy act. If the educator feels like humor in the video distracts in any way from the content, the best advice is just don't go there.

Stick to the Facts!

Bergmann and Sams (2012) also recommend not wasting student time with the lecture videos by talking about things that are not directly related to the learning objectives. Their example included an instructor talking about a favorite sports team in the video. There are other nursing-related aspects to this recommendation. Telling stories about patients you've encountered in clinical is a great teaching strategy, but one that should be saved for the in-class portion of time, not the videos. The patient stories you want to tell the students can be developed into great case studies for them to work on during the in-class time. Nursing students appreciate the cases that come from their educators' real-life experiences. They get to hear what really happened on the other end of the case study, which is sometimes not as real or meaningful when using a case study from a textbook. I rarely, if ever, use a case study that I have not developed myself. For one thing, I have lived these patient scenarios, and feel comfortable when the students ask me a question about patient history, for example. I know it, because I take care of these patients. I am of course very careful to use anonymous descriptions and many times change the storyline a bit to protect the anonymity of my patients. To reiterate, the information in the video should be directly related to the established learning objectives and in order to keep the video brief, should not be embellished with patient stories.

Different Ideas for Videos

When making lecture videos, most click through a shortened set of presentation slides previously developed for the class. Remember that the screen capture can be used in additional ways. As mentioned previously, a webcam can be used to record the instructor talking in the video, leaving out the slides altogether. A whiteboard with the screen capture can also be used for the off-load recording. Anything written on the board or typed on the computer will be recorded. Use of a concept map or an illustration to explain content to a student would be instances in which a whiteboard or document camera could be used.

Faculty can easily use the webcam to create their own whiteboard with a white sheet of paper. Simply point the webcam facing vertically down at a sheet of paper. Anything written on the paper will be captured by the webcam. It might help to check the orientation of the webcam prior to recording. The first time I used this technique, everything was recorded upside down. At times there is an important illustration or chart in the students' readings that the faculty might want to discuss for the video. Using the webcam facing downward toward readings or illustrations works very well without having to purchase additional expensive document cameras or other equipment. A video like this might also be used to teach the students how to do a concept map of their own, something educators use often within the face-to-face time. Of course, with a touch screen either on a computer or mobile device, a stylus can be used to write words or draw pictures on the screen while the video capture is recording. These provide some nice alternatives to using slides.

Another way to use screen capture would be to type notes within a word document as the educator discusses what is typed. Students seem to like this type of video and have stated it is easier for them to follow and pay attention to. Using a picture on the screen of the computer and the pointer to discuss points on the picture is a very effective way to make a video, as well. It is a great method for reviewing anatomy and physiology or parts of a physical assessment.

For example, when recording a video on the auscultation areas for the cardiac examination, a picture like the one shown in **Figure 6-3**, which I had drawn on my computer screen, was used. The screen capture video begins with a picture of only the skeleton. After a brief introduction of what the video will cover, the landmarks and abbreviations for the auscultation areas during a cardiac examination are taught one by one. For example, I teach where the angle of Louis is, what it means, and how it can be used to find other landmarks for the cardiac exam. Then show where the intercostal spaces are and how they are used as landmarks on the patients' chest to find the cardiac auscultation sites. Next comes a discussion about why the nurse should listen in certain areas, and use the cursor to point to each area with the computer arrow. Then create the circles on the video where

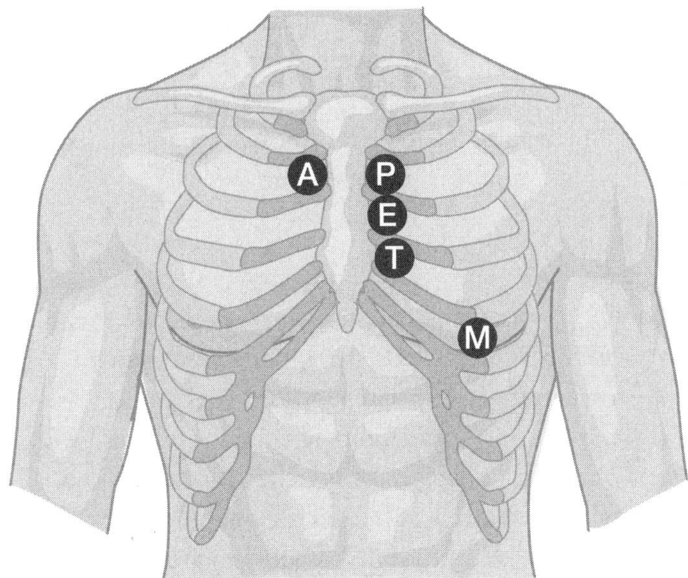

Figure 6-3 Cardiac examination picture.

each of the auscultation sites are as shown in Figure 6-3. Discuss as each is drawn what it is called and the exact location in terms of intercostal spaces and chest landmarks. Part of the students' assignment was to write up a quick note as they would in the patients' chart on a murmur they had "discovered" in the mitral area and bring it to class with them.

Bergmann and Sams (2012) have a wonderful idea to create the videos with another faculty member. When videos are done in this manner, the two faculty members can have a conversation about the content. Bergmann and Sams use the example of listening to a radio talk show. Very rarely do you just hear one person talking about a subject. Instead, the radio waves are populated with two, three, or even more people discussing one topic, each putting in their ideas, comments, and spin on the subject. Find an expert versed on a topic and use this type of recording as a video podcast (vodcast). Ask some questions of the expert, have them respond, and use the video as the learning modality for the students' offload. This is a great strategy for getting an expert opinion within your class without making the expert take a day out of their busy work week to come to your live class. As Bergmann and Sams have shown, this is an excellent way to make the video more fun for everyone.

Editing Your Video

As mentioned in a previous chapter, don't spend too much time editing the screen capture videos. Bergmann and Sams (2012) have suggested in their first flipped classroom text to add annotations, call outs, and zooming in and out within the videos. Annotations are written or typed and placed over the recorded video. They can be developed in numerous different shapes and sizes, and can be "dropped" into the video randomly. Call outs are very similar to annotations. A call out is described as a text box that will appear for a specified time in the video and go away as specifically timed during the editing process. The zoom feature within the screen capture software allows the video to zoom into a certain portion of the screen, and then zoom back out to the full screen to accent a certain area of the video. Bergmann and Sams have written that their students like these types of features because it does call attention to certain parts of the video and helps to keep the video a bit more entertaining.

It would be my recommendation to keep the videos very simple to begin with. Being realistic, it may take a bit of time to learn any new software. Recording a video can be extremely simple and fun to create. It really is as easy as clicking on the "GO" button, discussing the lecture points and then clicking on the "STOP" button. It doesn't get more simple than that! Adding some annotations, callouts, transitions, and zooming in later on when there is time is a great idea, because students do tend to like them.

Don't Forget About Copyright Laws

Bergmann and Sams (2012) bring up a very important point in their text about making videos on the computer. Be certain to keep everything within current copyright laws. Even though the videos will be used for educational purposes, there is the risk of violating copyright by using others' pictures, slides, and videos within the video. One option to avoid copyright laws for pictures is to draw your own on either paper or on the computer. If drawn on paper, a quick cell phone picture can be taken and turned into a PDF for sharing on the computer during the video. During the in-class activities, students will create some amazing work that applies to the content. It is very helpful for them to take a picture (or the educator can take one, too) and send it for posting on the learning management system for easy access by all. Educator drawings do not have to be perfect as long as they do the job of showing the students what is being discussed. When using a book picture with the webcam, be sure to reference the author of the text within the video. It would be the best idea not to use others' pictures, words, or work without consulting a copyright expert.

Sharing the Video With Students

When you are done recording your video, it is time to share it with the students. Depending upon which screen capture software used, there is a variety of ways to share videos. There are some websites that will store videos for a small fee and provide a link that can be sent to the students. There is also a way to load the video to the learning management Web-based system (such as Blackboard). Please contact the learning management system leaders or IT department for more information on how to do this within the learning management system (LMS). It may be that the IT department would rather the videos not be loaded into the LMS because they do take up quite a bit of space depending on the length of the video.

Another option for sharing videos with students would be to open a Google account and load the videos on YouTube within an "unlisted" setting. Anyone accessing and searching YouTube on the World Wide Web may watch your video if it is launched as public. There are some flipping instructors that have thousands of hits on their videos from people taking advantage of their knowledge on YouTube. This is quite a compliment to their work! If the video is launched as "private" each student will need to have a Google account and be invited by the faculty launching to view the video. Using the YouTube "unlisted" option is best if educators would rather the video not be able to be viewed by just anyone. The video can still be found within YouTube, but it is not easily searchable. When launching videos to a more public site, be extra cautious about not adding student and/or patient information that might be identifiable.

Another small but meaningful step to consider for the students when posting a video is to put the amount of time the video will run somewhere within the description. Students are appreciative of this little piece of information so that they can plan accordingly. For example, students may want to watch a video before they get supper on the table for their family but they only have 15 minutes to do so. Posting that the video runs about 12 minutes gives them enough information to know that they can watch the video during that time frame. Similarly, if the video is 20 minutes or maybe a smidge longer, the students know how much time they have to pencil in to get the video watched during their busy week.

When posting videos for students, it is also helpful to provide students with some information about how to watch and learn from the video. A discussion in class about faculty expectations is a great place to start, but could be followed by some simple instructions when posting the video, as well. It is also helpful to remind students of the learning objectives that are focused on the video in the instructions or description that accompanies the video. Any additional instructions can be related to faculty expectations for students as they watch the videos, but here are some basic instructions to consider:

1. The video is focused on (*topic of the video*) and will last approximately (*length of video*). The video will be focused on the following learning objectives (*insert the learning objectives*).

2. Please watch the video without any other distractions. Turn your cell phone on vibrate, turn off the television, and do not have additional screens open on your computer while viewing. Try to watch the video when you are not taking care of children or at work if at all possible.
3. It is best to complete all readings prior to watching the video.
4. You have an assignment that accompanies this video. Be sure to download, print, and have the handout ready to complete as you watch the video. *(if there is an accompanying assignment)*
5. Watch the video in an area that allows you to take some notes if possible.
6. Use the final instruction on the list to remind the students of any assignments that they will need to bring to the associated face-to-face class.

Adding instructions may seem fairly rudimentary, but it is a helpful step to clearly lay out expectations for students. When first flipping the classroom, the students need to have a bit more structure and direction in order for them to meet educator expectations.

Student Computer and Internet Access off Campus

It is not safe to assume that all students in the flipped classroom will have access to a computer with high-speed Internet at home. Particularly in some of the more rural areas, students can find watching even a short video challenging on a very slow Internet connection. There are a couple of solutions for this problem. One is to have students watch their videos while on campus within the library or in an on-campus computer lab. If they are far from campus, there is usually a public library nearby where they will have access to high-speed Internet and can watch their videos. Remind these students to take some earphones with them so they can hear the sound in the video without bothering other library patrons.

For the rare student who does not have access to a nearby public library, a copy of the video can be made either on a jump drive or compact disk (CD). Once all of the flipped videos are recorded for an entire class, the bookstore may be willing to sell a jump drive for the course with all the lectures preloaded on it for students in the class. Students would only be charged the cost of the jump drive, and could use this as a textbook purchase for financial aid. Students really like this idea. Negotiating with bookstores on how to get those videos preloaded on the jump drives and sell them as "new" even though they are "used" is the bigger challenge. In the meantime, when students want the videos on their jump drive, they can tell the educator. The videos can be loaded one at a time onto the student's personal jump drive very quickly. If the videos are short, they can also be emailed in a MP4 format for easy viewing. These steps only take a few minutes, and typically there are only one or two students who ask for the videos in this format. Because it is a little added time and effort on the part of the faculty member, reserve this extra step only for students who really need it. With students of different financial levels and geographic locations, educators need to be certain that the use of technology is not causing an additional barrier to student learning.

Using Others' Videos for Off-Load Content

With so many healthcare faculty across the nation and the world flipping the classroom, there is a paralleled explosion of video available for use on the Internet. There are many excellent and some not-so-excellent videos to choose from. These types of videos seem to help most with anatomy and physiology review and sometimes pathophysiology review. Unfortunately, nursing faculty may not find many videos online that are meeting the specific needs of nursing education. I tend to use most of my own videos for this reason. There are some great video sharing sites such as The Kahn Academy that are focused only on education, but have limited videos related to nursing topics at this time. Most of The Kahn Academy videos (at the time of this printing) have been about on K-12 learning. There has, however, been a recent call for nursing educators to begin posting their videos onto this sharing website. Therefore, perusing the videos on this type of educational website over time may become very fruitful. Perhaps some nurse educators reading this text will choose to load their nursing videos for widespread use on these websites in the future!

There are actually some very well-done videos on YouTube. However, getting to that one quality video takes quite a bit of video searching and viewing time. For these reasons, educators may save time and energy when they choose to screen capture their own videos. Nursing faculty know exactly what they want their students to learn. It will take a fraction of the time to just make a video instead of searching for hours to find one that may or may not fit the content to be taught. Some online videos at first glance seem to fit the content, but upon further viewing stray far away from the topic at hand. There are some additional cautions when using others' videos from Internet sources. There are some videos that seem to be great at first, but go sour as they go on. There are a few people who post to YouTube that use foul language or inappropriate humor in their videos that nursing educators do not want to endorse. To sum up, be cautious when assigning videos that are not self-created. On the other hand, watching a few videos from these sources can provide excellent ideas for educator-created recordings.

Other Ideas for Off-Load Materials

Although many educators using the flipped classroom model are doing so for the added benefit of delivering lecture through video, there are many other things that can be assigned as off-load content (see **Table 6-1** for examples). Some educators use these types of additional assignments on their own, while others use them in conjunction with a video to ensure that the students have viewed the video and will be prepared for the live class. One flipping colleague often uses what she has titled a "ticket to ride" assignment for her undergraduate pediatrics students. The ticket to ride can be any type of assignment that is connected to the video and must be completed during or after the video has been viewed. Once completed, the ticket to ride must be brought to class for entry into the face-to-face class activities. By requiring students complete a ticket to ride, the

Table 6-1 Off-Load Content

Off-Load Content	Description	Example
Faculty-Developed Video Lecture	Faculty-created video of lecture that they would have typically delivered in class	Lecture on cardiac physical assessment now condensed to 15–20 minute video that is posted for students to watch online prior to coming to class
Online Videos	Videos found on websites that are created by those other than the course faculty	The Kahn Academy videos YouTube videos (use caution)
Readings	Assigned readings	Textbooks Websites Evidence-based articles
Podcast	An audio recording of a lecture or similar content focused on learning objectives	Recording about essentials of cardiac assessment for nurses
Vodcast	A video recording of an instructor or other professional discussing content related to the learning objectives—very similar/same as video lectures	Lecture of an expert discussing the essentials of a cardiac assessment
Case Study	Written or video of simulated patient scenario	Presentation of a patient with cardiac symptoms for student to consider, perhaps answer questions about that are related to learning objectives
Worksheets	Pre-developed sheets with content for students to complete or fill in prior to coming to class	Worksheet developed around faculty-recorded video lecture to test knowledge or provide a learning assessment to gauge student preparedness for class
Discussion Questions	Questions related to the learning objectives asked to stimulate student thought, conversation, or debate	Set of discussion questions related to nursing care of cardiac patients or steps of cardiac assessment

(*Continues*)

Table 6-1 Off-Load Content (Continued)

Off-Load Content	Description	Example
Scavenger Assignment	Ask students to find an item to bring to the face-to-face class with them for discussion and further description.	While the student is in clinical, have them bring a copy of one of the policy/procedures from that unit to discuss in class. Is it evidence based? How can you tell?
Interview/Survey Gathering	Ask students to interview a certain population or take a survey—use specific guidelines and suggest ideas.	If studying theories, have students ask a nurse they know or one in clinical what theory they use the most with their patients. Discuss the responses in the face-to-face class time.
Student Reflective Journaling	Students are posed a question by faculty that they then write about in their personal reflective journal.	Faculty stimulate student thinking and reflection on current cases or scenarios that require inflection such as no-code status for cardiac patient with a pacemaker.
Observe and Report	Students observe behaviors or conduct, write it down, and report it to the class.	Students assigned to observe how many nurses and/or doctors wash hands prior to patient contact.
Learning Modules	Organized, paced learning materials that build upon one another and require student success on one portion prior to moving onto more complex material	Online case study that builds with questions for students to complete correctly prior to moving onto the next phase

faculty can be somewhat certain that the video has been watched by the students. Completing such an assignment can help each student be prepared to engage in the active learning activities planned for the in-class session.

Examples of "Ticket to Ride" and Other Off-Load Assignments

A simple worksheet for students to complete falls within the realm of the ticket to ride. Another idea is to ask the students to bring a summary of the video with them in a one-paragraph typed document. Similarly, assigning students to write a short summary of the top 3 things they found most important in the video recording can be helpful. Educators could also assign the beginning portion of a case study that will then unfold during the in-class time period. There are also other options, such as a simple vocabulary list. This assignment is helpful for students who are attempting to learn medical terminology needed for completion of a physical assessment. Asking each student to bring in 2 questions about the material to class that can lead the discussion during the in-class period is also an effective strategy.

Another idea for an off-load assignment is to ask each to bring to class the 3 most important nursing diagnoses for any kind of patient problem being studied, for example, congestive heart failure (CHF). For each of the nursing diagnoses the students develop, have them write about 2 or 3 important and associated nursing interventions. Have them include rationale for the 3 nursing diagnoses they've chosen as the most important. With all of the interventions that could possibly be associated with these 3 nursing diagnoses, why did they choose these specific interventions? The in-class activities that can flow from this type of off-load ticket to ride can then be reviewed during the in-class time and spur important conversations about nursing care and prioritization of diagnosis and interventions. For the advance practice students, the nursing diagnosis could be altered to include the top 3 differentials. For each of these differentials, have the students write about how to narrow down the diagnosis with further physical assessment and laboratory/diagnostic options. These can then be followed by the best ideas for a plan of care considering all other pieces of information about a patient presenting with signs and symptoms of CHF.

An additional idea for the ticket to ride could be a concept map. Have each student explain a disease process using their individual thought processes to connect a disease with the associated nursing interventions or plan of care. Many of the ticket-to-ride ideas listed here can be valuable off-load content to assign. It is important to remember, however, that the flipped classroom works best with a plan that allows students to work by themselves on the lower-ordered learning objectives and prepare themselves for more higher-ordered learning during the in-class time period.

Readings Assigned for Off-Load Content

Assignment of required and recommended readings are perhaps the most obvious idea for off-load content that is available. Even though the video is available for students, the readings do not go away and are still a valuable part of student preparation for in-class activities and learning overall. Testing to see if the students have completed the off-load readings may be desirable for educators who are concerned that their students might come to the in-class session unprepared. The online learning management system has been a valuable addition to off-load content for use with the flipped classroom for this reason. Faculty have used simple online quizzes that must be completed prior to coming to the in-class session. Faculty may consider tying these quizzes to the video created, but they could also be tied to the readings that are assigned as off-load as well.

Helping students self-regulate their needs for readings according to their level of understanding may help them manage their time reading more effectively. Students may not have the time and/or energy to read every word that assigned by their faculty. Students can learn to gauge what they need to read more about and what they feel knowledgeable about enough to not read at all. A good example lies within the physical assessment textbook assigned for undergraduate students. About one-fifth to one-third of each chapter is devoted to anatomy and physiology. There are some chapters that also focus a bit on pathophysiology. It is understandable that some of these topics in a physical assessment text are necessary to help students review and learn landmarks for how to complete assessments. But it is also a repeat of coursework that students have already mastered by passing pre-requisite courses. Nursing educators can help students differentiate their readings in order to augment what they already have learned, rather than feeling it necessary to read every word in the chapter.

A good example of differentiated reading could be a student that feels comfortable with his or her knowledge of anatomy, physiology, and pathophysiology of the cardiac system and vessels. The student can feel comfortable skipping the reading that reviews all of this content, moving on instead to the content that (s)he needs to gain knowledge about, the physical assessment information. When this idea is discussed with students, they often express relief. They begin to understand that they may not need to read every word about cardiac anatomy and physiology, but their fellow student very well may need that repetition because it was something that they didn't understand well in previous classes. When they get to the content on musculoskeletal, they may recognize that this was difficult subject for them in previous courses, and therefore will need to spend more time reviewing, reading, and studying that content than the next student may. Helping students to self-regulate their readings in this way can create a pattern of future self-regulation with the explosion of literature we are faced with in an evidence-based practice world.

In a graduate course, the nurse faculty may consider using "shared reading" assignments. For example, if there are 5 articles for assigned readings for an upcoming class, the reading responsibilities are shared among the students within a group. Consider that there are 15 students in the course. These 15 students could be split into groups of 5. Each student in the group of 5 takes responsibility for reading one article on the assigned reading list. Each student must create a bulleted outline and short summary about the article that the student reads and brings to class. The first 15 minutes of class is dedicated to the shared reading groups. The groups come together and the students hand out their outline/summary and spends a few minutes reviewing the article with those in their peer reading group. The idea to share responsibility came to me after participating in a hospital-based evidence practice group. The busy nurses on the evidence-based practice committee wisely shared their reading tasks. By doing so, each nurse was able to more fully read and analyze one or two articles in order to provide a nice summary for their peer group. It works beautifully and promotes group cohesiveness and accountability to complete assigned readings in a group fashion.

Learning Modules for Off-Load Content

Learning modules are wonderful off-load content for the flipped classroom. A learning module provides course materials to students in a logical, sequential order that guides them through content and assessments (University of Florida e-Learning, 2013). Instructors can use their imaginations to add text, pictures, quiz questions, and other materials together in a way that helps students step their way through content. Most learning modules are designed in such a way that requires students to master one section of material before moving onto the next section of material. Similarly, the materials in a learning module tend to build upon one another in a progressive fashion.

There are many ways to create learning modules that help students meet the lower-level learning objectives and prepare for the in-class activities. There are programs for purchase that make creating learning modules very easy. Many learning management systems have the capability for creating and launching learning modules. Educators can also create their own learning modules using a slide presentation program on their own computer. I have created a few learning modules using a simple case study that students click through on the presentation slides. The trick is to not allow them to move onto the next learning module content until they obtain the correct answer on the current slide. Most presentation programs have an option to shut off the ability to advance naturally to the next slide. On one slide, insert some material you want the student to learn with a button that can be clicked on to move to the next slide that has a quiz-type question. In the question slide, clickable buttons can be inserted that take the student to another slide that lets them move on (correct answer slide) or to an incorrect answer slide that makes them go back to the question until they select the correct answer. These modules are called *interactive PowerPoints*. My colleague Ann Henderson and I (Hessler & Henderson, 2013) did a study using these types of learning modules and found them to be extremely effective for student learning and fun as well. The only caveat is that the interactive PowerPoints do take a significant amount of time to develop.

Researching and Investigating Assigned for Off-Load Content

Embracing Prensky's (2010) idea of partnering with the students, allowing students to be more engaged with the development of their off-load content, can be quite useful. Students come up with some terrific ideas if given a chance. Using an off-load assignment that asks students to investigate and research a topic allows them to be creative. While teaching a course that focused on the professorial role for nurse educators, I created an off-load assignment for students to interview a current faculty member about tenure. There were very few guidelines for the assignment other than to ask a faculty member who is on the tenure track to share his or her thoughts about the tenure process. In addition to the interview, I asked the students to either support or refute their interviewee's comments with two to three references. During the live class, the students were asked if their interviewee had mostly positive or mostly negative ideas/thoughts about the tenure process. After splitting into two groups, a discussion about the main positive and negative comments with associated literature sources ensued. At the end of class, each of the groups reported to one another, including the references that they had found in the process. The conversation around the tenure process was very real and lively, and pulled in evidence that the students found on their own rather than having it as assigned readings.

Students can be assigned to an investigation in the off-load for many different topics. If the learning objectives point to population-based health, have students pick a population to investigate. Provide some general guidelines for the assignment, but also allow enough flexibility for students to be self-driven and investigate a population that is of particular interest to them. These types of assignments meet the learning objectives while simultaneously allowing for an element of student passion. An example might be when the learning objectives are focused on politics and legislation. Have the students find a bill that they can report about to the class. If the learning objectives are focused on patient use of alternative therapies, have the students individually or in small groups choose a therapy to investigate. If learning about community resources, send students out to investigate what is available in their own community and what that resource offers. Culture, health disparities, and disease states are some other examples of how to send the students on a treasure hunt to meet the learning objectives of the off-load content.

Differentiated Off-Load Assignments—Mastery Learning?

The idea of mastery learning as described in the discussions of Bergmann and Sams (2012, 2014) and Bretzmann (2013) is an idea that has been introduced, but not embraced widely in nursing education. Although mastery learning was first introduced around the 1920s, it gained popularity when reintroduced by Benjamin Bloom of Bloom's Taxonomy. Mastery learning is described by Ben Johnson on Edutopia (Johnson, 2013) as students mastering certain concepts and skills before moving onto additional concepts and skills. If students do not master the skill or concept, they must stay within the current step until it is mastered. Students move through content and "master" the learning objectives at their own pace. Bergmann and Sams go on to further describe the key components of mastery learning to include: students working either by themselves or in small groups at their own pace; instructor using formative assessment as students progress through learning objectives; and students not mastering the learning objectives receiving remediation until able to master them.

In most of the nursing courses, the assessment of mastery comes with a test or exam to determine whether each individual student has learned the content and is ready to move on to the next content within a course. In the framework of mastery learning, testing should be only one of the elements of assessing mastery of content. Think of a student who has done poorly on one or two exams, but well on a few others. They end up with an average of exam grades that allows a student to pass the course, but not necessarily reach the point of mastery with all of the content within. Similarly, think of a student who fails the first exam in the course. Should this student be allowed to continue on in the course regardless of this lack of mastery? It leaves an important educational question left unanswered– Where is the *remediation* to reach mastery in nursing education?

Although some nursing education studies have shown positive student outcomes when mastery learning is implemented (Sutton Roberts, Ingram, Flack, & Jones Hayes, 2013) it is not often used due to the difficulty associated with implementation. Bergmann and Sams (2012) have described how they've used mastery learning within their high school flipped classroom quite successfully. In their class, students are busy and engaged in their own learning doing asynchronous activities within the classroom. They organize their students at the beginning of each class, and know which students need to work at which levels. They describe talking to every student, in every class, every day. Is nursing education ready for this type of asynchronous activity within the classroom? With the current paradigm of teaching, learning, and assessment in nursing education, it seems like a daunting task. However, thinking of mastery learning within the off-load materials might seem more manageable.

Mastery learning applied to off-load materials has the potential to develop self-regulation of learning among nursing students. The previous discussion of how to decrease a current 3-hour lecture period into a smaller off-load video lecture in order to not repeat anything in the video leaves a great deal of room for mastery learning. One might consider assigning the off-load materials similarly to how textbooks and other references have been assigned within a syllabus. There are some materials that could be required to be watched or reviewed prior by every student prior to coming to class, while other materials are listed as recommended. The recommended materials focus on each individual student's understanding of content from previous classes.

Using cardiac physical assessment as an example, pages of reading in the cardiac assessment chapter that are focused on the learning objectives for completion of the physical assessment could be listed as required reading. The additional pages of the chapter could be assigned as recommended depending on individual student needs for review/reading. The recommended pages are focused on content that students have had in previous courses. Videos can be assigned in a similar way. Those videos that are directly related to what will be discussed in class could be listed as required viewing. However, those videos that are mainly review of anatomy and physiology or some other content that students have had in previous course work could be labeled as recommended.

At first, nursing students have difficulty with this type of mastery concept. They may be tempted to watch and read everything for fear that they will be somehow fall behind or miss something. But soon students realize that their off-load materials can be as little or as much as work as they need them to be in order to meet the learning objectives. Here is where the mastery learning becomes part of the off-load process. It could be described as differentiated reading and viewing, an idea that parallels the idea of mastery learning. In this paradigm, students understand that they are adult learners in control of their own time. Teaching students how to manage their time in order to complete necessary material with review if necessary has been a big part of my flipped classroom framework.

Conclusion

The idea of off-load material within the flipped classroom can be focused on many different teaching and learning modalities to help students master the lower-level objectives within the flipped classroom model. Although the recent ability to record lectures on video and provide them to students online has been a big part of the definition of the flipped classroom, it is not the only way to assign off-load content. As nurse educators begin to think about how to assign off-load content, they need to be creative. Think of things that are readily applicable and tangible or concrete for student learning. Exposure to fellow flipping faculty who can augment ideas and provide inspiration for the growth of new ones can be extremely helpful and inspiring. Partnering with students to involve them in the assignment of off-load assignments is a challenge, but is productive for both parties. Nurse educators may be very surprised at students' ability to develop very meaningful assignments that are directly related to both learning the objectives and individual passions in nursing. It is okay to use the same off-load content over and over within the same course until new ideas come to mind. The one caveat is that any off-load assignment should be directly related to the learning done within the face-to-face class. As new ideas begin to flow, each nurse educator will be surprised at how meaningful these off-load assignments will become.

References

Benner, P. (2001). *From novice to expert: Excellence and power in clinical nursing practice.* Upper Saddle River, NJ: Prentice-Hall.

Bergmann, J., & Sams, A. (2012). *Flip your classroom: Reach every student in every class every day.* Eugene, OR: International Society for Technology in Education.

Bergmann, J., & Sams, A. (2014). *Flipping learning: Gateway to student engagement.* Eugene, OR: International Society for Technology in Education.

Bretzmann, J. (2013). *Flipping 2.0: Practical strategies for flipping your class.* New Berlin, WI: The Bretzmann Group.

Hessler, K., & Henderson, A. (2013). Interactive learning research: Application of cognitive load to nursing education. *International Journal of Nursing Education Scholarship, 10*(1), 133–141.

Johnson, B. (2013). *Using mastery learning for success with difficult students.* Retrieved from http://www.edutopia.org/blog/mastery-learning-success-difficult-students-ben-johnson

Prensky, M. (2010). *Teaching digital natives: Partnering for real learning.* Thousand Oaks, CA: Corwin SAGE.

Sutton Roberts, D., Ingram, R. R., Flack, S. A., & Jones Hayes, R. (2013). Implementation of mastery learning in nursing education. *Journal of Nursing Education, 52*(4), 234–237.

Swellar, J., van Merrienboer, J., & Paas, F. (1998). Cognitive architecture and instructional design. *Educational Psychology Review, 10*(3), 251–296.

University of Florida e-Learning. (2013). *Learning modules.* Retrieved from https://lss.at.ufl.edu/help/Learning_Modules

CHAPTER 7

Now What? How to Manage Your Class Time Effectively in the Flipped Model of Learning

Introduction

The Intentional Instruction Model describes the live, face-to-face class time with the term: *In-Class Activities* (see **Figure 7-1**). As previously described, the in-class activities should be targeted to teach higher-ordered learning objectives. Ideally, each in-class activity should build upon the off-load assignments. Some faculty spend a small amount of class time to determine if students have completed off-load assignments. Doing so can help to insure that students are ready to fully participate during the in-class activities. Similarly, some educators have changed their syllabus or grading policy to include points for both off-load assignments and in-class activities. Strategies for evaluation of learning in the flipped classroom vary depending on educator preference. Evaluation of learning in the flipped classroom is more fully discussed in Chapter 8.

It seems that much of the clamor surrounding the flipped classroom has focused on newly available technology to record and move lectures from the group to the individual setting. With so much emphasis within the flipped classroom on the technology, it may be easy to forget about the importance of the in-class time. Many would argue that the most meaningful benefit of the flipped

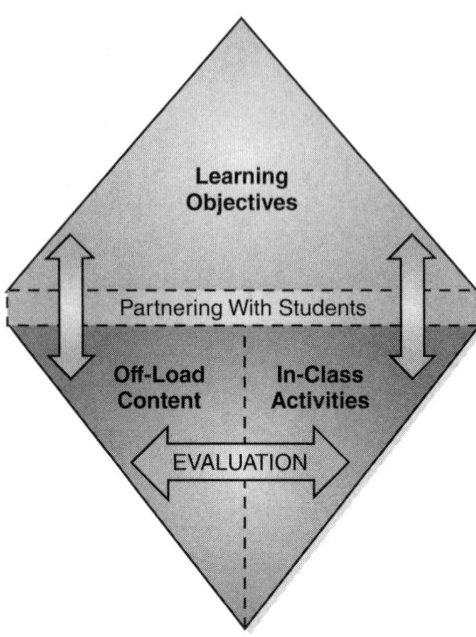

Figure 7-1 Intentional Instruction Model.

classroom for nursing faculty lies in the capability to use the entire face-to-face time with students for active, individualized teaching. But re-conceptualizing the live class time with students could be a daunting task for some nurse educators. Some may have the remaining question, "If lecture is not used during the live class, what will the students do?" The answer to this question is extremely exciting: They will be learning nursing concepts on a deeper level. How to successfully structure this deeper, more meaningful in-class learning experience is the focus of this chapter.

The term *active learning* has been floating around nursing education for the last several decades, but what does it really mean? Active learning is described as an educational approach in which the instructor has students apply content during instructional activities and reflect upon the actions that they have taken (Thomas, 2009). Active learning often has the student in the roles of problem solver, team member, peer reviewer, and/or teacher. Active learning does require students to function at a high cognitive level because they analyze, synthesize, and evaluate (Thomas, 2009). Being student-centered, active teaching strategies require students to take an active role in their own learning. When such strategies are used, students must be physically and mentally present in order to engage their brain and truly learn the content. When it comes to active learning, there may be more than meets the eye. Some teaching activities masquerade as active when in fact they do not require students to function at a higher level of learning. One example is gaming, which requires rote memorization regurgitation from individual students rather than a deeper learning of the content. The in-class time is precious, and should be reserved for those activities that truly require students to apply content learned in the off-load setting in a meaningful way.

Some recent research comparing an active learning environment to that of straight lecture in nursing education did show positive results. Shin, Sok, Sun Hyun, and Ja Kim (2014) formed a research partnership between Seoul, South Korea and Chicago nurse researchers to design a descriptive, cross-sectional comparative design with 147 senior nursing students. About half of the students were taught with active teaching strategies, including high-fidelity simulation, situation-based case studies, standardized patients, audio-video playback, reflective activities, and technology-based learning programs. The other half of students were taught using what was described as traditional lecture. The Korean Nurses' Core Competency Scale was used to measure each participant's core competency level. The scale contained 70 items and 5 subdomains that measured human understanding and communication, professional attitudes, critical thinking and evaluation skills, general nursing performance (such as physical assessment and medication administration), and special nursing performance (such as critical care scenarios). Overall scores and nursing competency assessments were significantly higher for students who had been exposed to active learning than those who were taught with lecture. Students were also asked to self-evaluate their learning achievement and satisfaction in the course, with the active learning group scoring these items higher than their lecture counterparts. The study is added here to lend credibility to the active learning recommended as part of the flipped classroom. Although this study did not focus on the flipped classroom, it does show clearly that active learning creates a more rounded nursing student. It is difficult to argue with the results of such a well-designed and thorough study conducted by our Korean colleagues.

Certainly there are some nurse educators reading this chapter that have been using active learning within their classrooms for quite some time. These types of educators may experience an easier transition from straight lecture in their teaching repertoire to the flipped classroom. Flipped learning has at its core active learning within the classroom. It is understandable that nurse educators who have been using active learning strategies in the classroom all along might not see anything different about flipped learning. It is true that the interactive teaching and learning strategies are not as innovative as the ability to provide lecture as "homework" to be viewed prior to class. However, even educators familiar with the use of interactive learning activities can admit the advantage of more time for them when the flipped classroom is implemented.

When re-conceptualizing the face-to-face time with students, it may help educators to think of the flipped classroom as another way to mix lecture with active learning. Lecture does not go away in the flipped classroom model of teaching. Instead, it shrinks to the sideline as active learning takes the spotlight. The nursing classroom of the past may have had lecture as the main teaching strategy with use of active learning as a secondary method. But the flipped classroom allows more time to engage students with interactive teaching strategies instead of leaving them to function as a smaller piece of the pedagogy puzzle. Active learning strategies were likely always on the in-class menu, but used mostly as a dessert. When the flipped classroom is used, the teaching menu lists active learning as the main meal. Lecture is still on the menu, but is used as a before-meal appetizer.

Ideas for active learning during the in-class time created by the flipped classroom pedagogy are truly endless, limited only by educator imagination. Admittedly, coming up with these creative ideas to engage students in active learning is easy for some and difficult for others. Sharing ideas with other faculty members (some nursing faculty and some from other professions) can be extremely helpful to expand the active learning horizons. Listening to other educators' in-class ideas offers fuel for the imagination. Many active learning strategies are not content dependent. Translation of active learning strategies can therefore take place. Attending conferences, reading articles, and starting a flipping group of faculty on campus are some ways to get exposure to the most innovative ideas for in-class activities. Keeping a "flipping journal" is also a valid suggestion. Too often, an idea comes to mind that all too suddenly slips right back out again before it can fully develop. For this reason, use of a cellphone notebook or mobile device to leave little notes about in-class ideas is beneficial. Some ideas are brilliant and work out splendidly. Others end up in the recycle bin. All in all, the students are likely to appreciate the additional educator effort and imagination required to make their learning environment more meaningful, even if 100% success is not always possible.

The goal of this chapter is to assist in the reconceptualization of in-class time with tips and ideas for the development of an individualized flipped classroom. Helping educators to structure the in-class learning time for optimal student engagement will be discussed. Some of the common challenges and associated solutions that may arise with use of the flipped classroom will be reviewed. The discussion includes examples of the most commonly used in-class activities applied to the nursing education flipped classroom.

The Flipped Classroom In-Class Structure

Different educators conceptualize their flipped classroom in-class time in different ways. Educators are themselves unique individuals, each of whom brings a different flavor to their teaching style. The same is true with the different approaches to the flipped classroom. A more "free-spirited" faculty member may feel very comfortable with a level of chaos in their classroom, while the more "type A" faculty member may find that more structure in the classroom is a must. Now take into account that students in the class have as many different personalities and learning styles as there are names on the roster. The attempt to please everyone during the in-class time is tempting, but not terribly realistic. What seems to be more consistent is student appreciation for structure in the classroom from one class to the next overall. It is recommended that the in-class learning time within the flipped classroom model have a consistent and reliable structure from one class to another for the entire semester.

Although organizing the in-class time for the flipped classroom must come from individual preference, there are some solid ideas for the flipped classroom structure that have been successful for educators from all different sorts of professions. Bergmann and Sams (2012) serve as the first example in their pioneer text on flipped learning. When flipping the classroom within a high school–level advanced placement chemistry class, the authors opened their live class with a warmup activity lasting about 5 minutes including attendance (see **Figure 7-2**). Next was a question and answer period directed at the offload materials assigned that lasted approximately 10 minutes. The rest of the class time (about 75 minutes) they called "guided and independent practice." The focus of this time was spent on a packet of practice problems, experiments, examples from the instructor as well as the students, and depending on their schedule, a lab day.

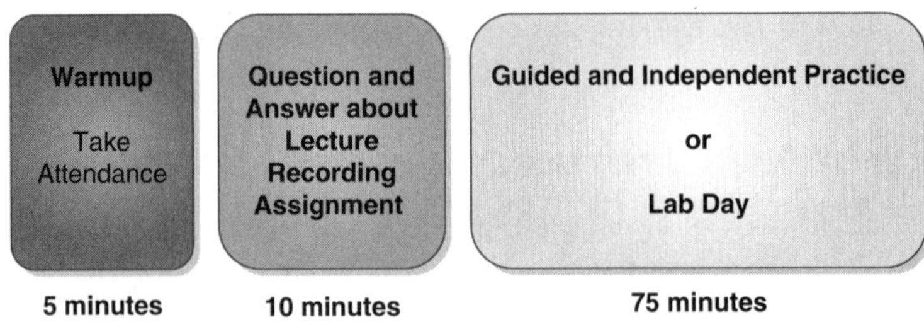

Figure 7-2 Bergmann and Sams' flipped classroom template.

When students were working through the problems or on assigned experiments, the instructors were able to move through the classroom to help where help was needed. Those students who comprehended the material and were working a bit more independently had access to an answer guide for self-grading. Within this model, the instruction was focused around the students and not the teacher. The teacher's role in the flipped classroom was no longer to deliver information to the students. Instead, the teachers transitioned to the role of resident experts, available to assist with specific and individual learning needs (Bergmann & Sams).

Flipping a nursing education classroom should have a similar and consistent structure throughout the entire course. Flipping the classroom is very likely a new pedagogy for the students to get used to. As previously discussed, this type of educational change can be difficult and bring about a certain amount of mistrust and resistance from the students. Offering a consistent structure for students to rely upon when the class is flipped has the potential to decrease their natural tendencies toward anxiety and resistance to the pedagogy. A set class structure can take the fear of the unknown largely out of the resistance equation, and set up a level of trust between faculty and students. Implementing the in-class time within a structure can provide consistency for faculty, as well. Within a structure, time can flow as necessary between any planned learning activities. Following Bergmann and Sams' (2012) example, nurse educators can develop their own structure that fits their personality, teaching style, learning objectives, and student needs in their respective flipped classrooms.

Opening the Live Class

What is the best way to start or open the in-class portion of the flipped classroom? There are a number of possibilities to consider. By now we understand that learning within the flipped classroom actually begins with assigning students a variety of off-load materials. Many educators considering the flipped classroom have a common and valid concern that students will not access the off-load materials as assigned and therefore will not be prepared for the in-class activities. One of the strategies to assist with this potential problem is an assessment of off-load learning assigned. When such an assessment or evaluation of learning is used, the in-class time often opens with students taking a short quiz, presenting assigned materials, or hand in worksheets or other assignments prior to the planned learning activities.

Class can also be opened with a question and answer (Q & A) period about the off-load materials assigned. Assessment of student readiness for class and the Q & A period can be tied together. This may be the most useful approach to beginning each flipped classroom, in my opinion. Students are assigned to bring one or two questions about the off-load material to class after completing all off-load materials (reading and lecture video). Students must hand in their questions in hard copy to the instructor when they enter the class. During the Q & A, students ask the questions they've developed. It is common for students to have similar questions. For this reason, the Q & A does not take as much time as one might think. This type of assignment not only confirms that each student has at the very least accessed the off-load materials, but also stimulates an in-depth discussion about the materials reviewed at home.

When opening class in this way, there is not a need for the nurse educator to grade any additional off-load assignments. Some students have voiced that they had no questions about the off-load materials and therefore brought nothing to class. Of course there are two realities, either they really did understand everything or they did not complete or access the off-load materials at all. As a result, an additional assignment for students is to write down and bring to class two points of the off-load material that they felt were the most important, including a short rationale of why. These salient points are called "take-home points." With this approach, students must bring *something* to the live class that can help to stimulate the discussion about the materials and show faculty that they have accessed and viewed the off-load assignments. Some students will bring questions, while others will bring their most important points to the discussion. It is only required that they bring either questions or take-home points, but students often bring both to the live class.

Some faculty open their flipped classroom with a quiz to assess learning of the off-load materials and student readiness for the live class. The quiz is typically short in nature (about 10 to 15 short questions) and can be handwritten or electronic. Some educators use a classroom response system with clicker questions for students as a strategy to assess learning of off-loads materials at the beginning of the flipped class. The one advantage to the classroom response system is the self-grading capability. The handwritten quizzes need to be graded by educators. A similar strategy is to use a short online quiz that students must complete prior to coming to class within the existing learning management system (such as Blackboard, for example). The learning management system may also allow for mastery of the content through quizzing. Each student may need to earn a certain score on the quiz prior to being marked as complete.

To summarize, the beginning of the flipped classroom template should be developed to include a Q & A period in which students can clear up any questions they have about the off-load materials. Whether done in conjunction with or independent of an off-load learning assessment is the choice of the instructor. Time allotted to the Q & A will fluctuate from class to class depending on student needs, but a general timeline should be established by the faculty member in the attempt to keep class on track as much as possible. An estimated time of 15 minutes at the beginning of the class for the Q & A is usually sufficient. The first few times the classroom is flipped, keep track of how long the Q & A period lasts. This information can be used for future planning for the same flipped class.

In-Class Active and Interactive Learning Activities

Once the flipped classroom in-class session is opened with the Q & A or evaluation of student off-load learning session, the active learning typically follows. The exact development of these activities will depend on the topic, associated learning objectives, and time available within the live class. There are many excellent active learning activities for the nurse educator to use for the in-class session of the flipped classroom. The possibilities of what to do with class time are too expansive to include and adequately describe within the pages of this book. Included will be an overview of the most useful activities for use in nursing education. For those looking for more ideas, reading a book that is specifically focused on active learning is an excellent idea. Doing so can lead to more and more creative ideas of how the in-class time can be used effectively for active student learning.

To Group or Not to Group?

There exists some debate among flipping educators about having students work in groups or individually during in-class learning time. It is likely as one gains more experience with flipping the classroom, that some of each will be used. Additional debate surrounding group membership and selection to achieve the best student learning outcomes exists. Should students work in the same groups all semester to create a group cohesiveness and consistency? Should the group membership be changed every week to expose students to more individual views and personalities? Should students be allowed to self-select group members or should they be assigned? Although cooperative learning has been examined in the nurse education literature, many of these questions have remained largely unanswered.

Austria, Baraki, and Doig (2103) conducted an interpretive descriptive qualitative inquiry to explore student nurse and patient experiences when collaborative learning was used during a clinical experience. The sample consisted of 11 first-semester baccalaureate nursing students assigned to pairs to provide care on an inpatient surgical oncology unit. Assuming that learning has a social component, the authors theorized that student behavior and performance would be influenced by this collaborative approach to clinical learning. The purposes provided for use of student dyads included enhancement of learning with peer collaboration, an answer to scarcity of clinical placements for students, and the ability to more closely supervise and teach students during the clinical course.

For two consecutive days, the student dyads worked together but with clear role delineation assigned by the clinical instructor. The first day, one student would complete the physical assessment and direct patient care. The other was assigned to be a partner in data gathering, decision making, and implementation of nursing care. The following day, the roles were reversed. Themes that emerged from student informants included a sense of support, decrease in anxiety, and an increase in confidence to care for patients using the dyad approach. The theme of increased efficiency was also discussed, because the two students helped one another complete necessary nursing interventions during the clinical day. Patient participants felt the student dyads were thorough, attentive, caring, and approachable, but at times overwhelming (Austria et al., 2013).

Researchers in this study recognized that although collaborative learning does aim to provide a sense of equality with shared goals, some students naturally assume more responsibility while others are more passive (Austria et al., 2013). Due to this natural occurrence, the authors recommended clear guidelines and assignments when collaborative learning is used. Orienting students to the collaborative process was also recommended. These recommendations seem easy to implement and have the potential to make group work more meaningful.

In Canada, a study conducted by Trueman, Osuji, and El-Hussein (2014) yielded interesting results. In this study, student pairs were assigned their own patient, but were instructed to come together

Table 7-1 BSN Students Experiences With Dyadic Learning

Themes	Corresponding Subthemes	Take-home Ideas
Work Engagement	• Collaboration • Interpersonal relationships • Partnership	Dyads can create a positive state of mind characterized by dedication. Students learn to work with others to negotiate patient care and outcomes.
Relational Practice	• Interpersonal relationships • True partnership • Feeling of comfort • Facilitates learning	Dyadic learning provides specific social support that decreases student stress and increases self-efficacy.
Autonomy	• Improves practice • Enhanced communication • Enhanced critical thinking • Opportunity to hone team attitudes	Autonomy can be explored when working with others. Self-confidence slowly increases as students are able to learn together what they will soon do on their own.
Empowerment	• Knowing your dyad makes a difference • Knowledge expansion • Overcome challenges • Learn about own weaknesses	Dyadic learning provides a safe environment for students to recognize and share strengths and weaknesses through consultation and collaboration experiences.

Developed with information from Trueman, G., Osuji, J., & El-Hussein, M. T. (2014). Baccalaureate nursing students' experience of dyadic learning in an acute care setting. *Journal of Nursing Education, 53*(9), S65–S72.

to discuss the patients, assessments, and nursing care throughout the clinical day. Using a phenomenological approach, student participants' reflective journals were reviewed for themes. After data analysis, overall themes included work engagement, relational practice, autonomy, and empowerment (see **Table 7-1**). Students reported feeling more confident in their care decisions when working with a student partner. Researchers commented on student dyad ability to quickly communicate and streamline care when required to work together. The dyadic learning provided students with a specific sort of social support that alleviated stress and promoted psychological and professional well-being. The ability to bounce ideas and thoughts off of a peer can be an invaluable part of student learning. It also simulates how nurses conduct business on a daily basis. Creating a culture in which students see consultation as a natural part of their work process may encourage more collaboration in the nursing care setting. In this study, the ability to work in pairs was linked to an increase in self-efficacy as well (Trueman et al., 2014).

When groups are used in the flipped classroom, they should be used with clear direction from the educator. Perhaps dividing the work ahead of time and assigning pieces to each group member would be a helpful approach to addressing the natural tendencies of dominant and submissive personalities. The idea of individualized assignments for each group member in the off-load coupled with collaboration sessions during the in-class time could address these tendencies. The work of the group is more likely to be evenly distributed if assigned by the educator. Each student within the group may be able to contribute on a more meaningful level as well. This type of collaborative learning is used with the *"Expert of the Day"* in-class activity (to read more about this activity, see the "Problem-based Learning" section later in this chapter).

Gagnon and Roberge (2011) conducted qualitative research investigating nursing students' experiences with group work. The 96 nursing student participants were either in their first or third semester of the nursing program. Students were asked to describe their experience of the process of working in a group as fully as they could. It was found that the most occurring theme students shared focused on the coordination element of group work. Students discussed with the researchers that their main difficulty with group work was finding a common meeting time and place to complete it. Also included in this theme were student difficulties with transportation to group work meetings. Students shared their appreciation of having time in class to complete group work. The flipped classroom allows for group work during the scheduled class time. Flipping essentially resolves the main student concerns found in this study revolving around group work. It also supports student learning and participation in group work, because the instructor is working with each group periodically throughout the in-class session. These aspects of the flipped classroom allow for promotion of student group learning in very significant ways.

In the same study, the more shy students reported feeling a greater sense of assertiveness when in a smaller group (Gagnon & Roberge, 2011). As a result, they were more comfortable expressing their opinions and being a part of the group processes. Clear communication, cooperation, and mutual respect among group members were also common themes. Not surprisingly, some students preferred to complete work alone while others preferred the group setting. These results further support the assignment of individual tasks assigned as off-load assignments, then bringing individual work to the in-class session for group assembly and collaboration. This sort of strategy also more readily mirrors similar settings of group work in practice settings, such as evidence-based practice and research councils. As the authors state, group work can serve as a conduit for positive learning environments (Gagnon & Roberge, 2011). At the same time, attention of faculty to findings of such research considering student concerns about group work should be considered when developing collaborative learning environments.

Kung's (2013) writing regarding group work in college mathematics may be helpful for nurse educators to review as they are considering similar strategies in their higher education settings. Knowing the research about student group work is largely positive, Kung has provided some research-based ideas about key ingredients in the promotion of successful student group work. Student group work must include clear group goals and individual accountability. Consider how these two necessary ingredients of successful group work can be fostered by a faculty member. Use of individual assignments for each member of a group and creating a clear goal for group work ahead of time are plausible approaches. Use of a pre-developed group work guide can provide this structure as well as consistency for group work each time it is assigned. Creating such a template for students to help guide their work within the group can help students stay on

NURS 645 – GROUP ACTIVITY SHEET

DATE: ____________ GROUP MEMBERS: ______________________________

Record Keeper: ____________________ Spokesperson: ____________________

Time:	Task:
10 minutes	Review Group Assignment (Handed out during class)
10 minutes	Assign Tasks 1. 2. 3. 4.
20 minutes	Complete Assigned Tasks
15 minutes	Group Collaboration Time • Each member report • Discuss collective thoughts • Complete a summary
5 minutes	Review and Reflect: • Did the group answer questions with research-based answers? • Group process—Did the group agree on collective topics?

Figure 7-3 Group work template.

task and create a structure for their group process. **Figure 7-3** is a template that can be altered depending on educator and course needs.

Answers to the many questions surrounding group work in the flipped classroom may be different for different educators. Assigning groups is preferred by many educators due to undesirable experiences with self-select student groups. When self-selection of groups is allowed, the students who naturally congregate together outside of class as friends have a tendency to end up in the class groups together. The situation then arises when the group ends up chatting and laughing more than actually working and learning. Group self-selection also has the potential to create an uncomfortable segregation of sorts among students within the classroom. In addition to these considerations, it is a reality that nurses cannot choose whom they work with on a daily basis in the practice setting. Assigning student groups therefore more closely represents their future work setting as a nurse.

Some faculty allow a trial of student self-selection to groups. Evidence that the students' self-selected groups function in an appropriate manner and work well together will lead to continued self-selection. However, if there are problems with self-selection during the first assignment, the faculty member can then assign the groups as an alternative method. Many educators might agree that self-selection of groups has worked well with some cohorts of nursing students and terribly with others. The personalities that come together in any given group of nursing students can be either conducive or restrictive to self-selection of work group members. For this reason, a trial of allowing self-selection may give the students a bit more freedom and comfort in the group work process.

How many students should be in each group is another question up for debate. It may depend on what type of material is being taught to the students. Through much trial and error, it is my experience that smaller groups work the best for the in-class time of the flipped classroom. The maximum number of students in a group for best group process has been about three to five within the same group. Smaller groups tend to keep every student engaged in the content. Each student opinion is more likely to be shared with the group within the time allotted for any given exercise in the smaller group as well. When the groups get larger, there always seem to be some students working and some not engaged or feeling that they cannot help due to the dominance of the "worker bees" assigned to their group.

Thought Partner

An alternative to having students work in larger groups is the use of a consistent "thought partner" (see **Figure 7-4**). The "thought partner" is a great strategy that originated from an esteemed colleague, Dr. Kathleen Dunemn. Having an extensive career in the military prior to coming to nursing education, Dr. Dunemn has brought with her some excellent critical thinking strategies that engage and stimulate thought among members of a group. Having a "thought partner" is one of these strategies. Supported by research (Austria et al., 2013; Trueman et al., 2014) dyad learning has many distinct advantages. At the beginning of the class, the idea of a thought partner is explained thoroughly to the students, including how the dyad will be used throughout the semester. Then the students are asked to choose a thought partner on their own.

The strategy of allowing students to choose their own thought partner is based on the thought that in nursing practice, thought partners are not assigned but naturally emerge from practice settings. Once students choose a thought partner, that dyad stays the

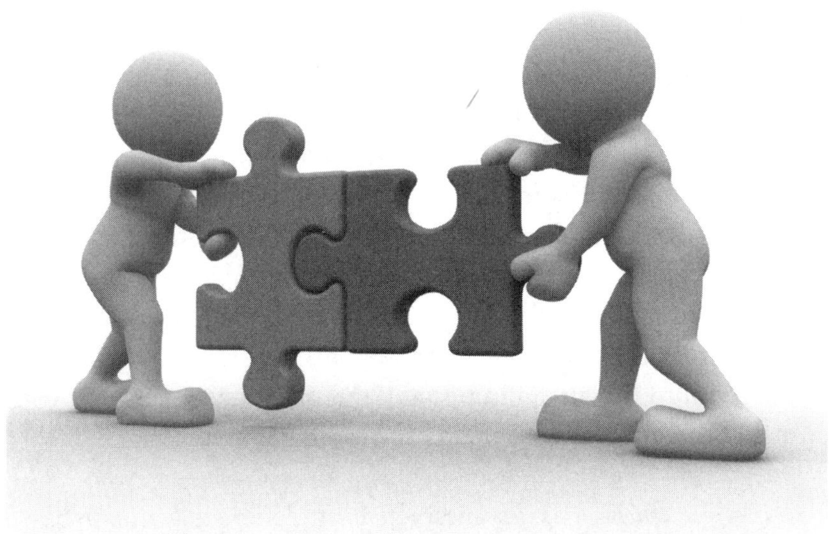

Figure 7-4 Thought partner.

same for the remainder of the class. The only exception would be the unusual development of an obvious or unmanageable personality conflict between the two students. Thankfully this happens very rarely. During the active learning sessions, students are often assigned to pair up with their thought partner to think about, discuss, and produce an opinion or recommendation related to a discussion question or debate topic.

The above strategy is similar to the "think-pair-share" strategy that is often used in interactive lecture-based or active learning activities within the classroom. Students are first asked to "think" about a question or concept on their own for a specified period of time after which they turn to their neighbor to "pair" and then "share" the ideas and thoughts developed during the "think" time period. Typically, a few student pairs are then asked to share their thoughts with the entire classroom, which serves once again to stimulate discussion and deeper thought from the entire group. To take it one step farther, the dyads (or thought partners, if using that strategy) can also pair with another dyad to discuss in a group of four the topic at hand.

Mini-Lecture

Often educators who are assisting students in group activities find that similar questions come forth from students about the case or content from one group to the next. A "mini-lecture" is a great additional teaching strategy to address a reoccurring question throughout the groups in the classroom. A mini-lecture is described as a brief and focused lecture to the entire class about a topic of confusion or content in need of clarification. Drawing the student attention from their group work back to the attention of the expert faculty member in the room to explain an important and often misunderstood concept is also described with the term "just-in-time teaching."

Just-in-time teaching is an interactive student engagement-based pedagogy that takes into consideration the level of student learning that has already occurred and where it is in need of augmentation by the instructor (Novak, 2014). In higher education, just-in-time teaching can be used in a couple of different ways. Providing a mini-lecture for teaching content that everyone in the class has the potential to benefit from is using just-in-time teaching. The pedagogy can also be used after evaluating student understanding of off-load materials prior to designing in-class activities, assignments, and/or lecture materials. In either instance, the main idea of just-in-time teaching is to reach a specific group of students at their specific level of understanding about the content rather than providing a blanketed approach to the student audience that attempts to catch those who know little as well as those who know much. Just-in-time teaching is another strategy that swings the educational pendulum back toward individualized student learning needs.

Case-Based Learning

Case studies have been used by nurse educators for years, but have not been researched heavily in the field of nursing education (Day, 2011). According to Billings and Halstead (2005), a case study is defined as the in-depth analysis of a true-to-life clinical situation used to illustrate course concepts. The case study applies the didactic content and theory to a real-life scenario, more recently referred to as a low-fidelity simulation. The case study allows students to practice making decisions and explore alternate types of thinking (Purtee, Ulloth, & Caputi, 2005). Students learn about treatment options and are able to evaluate their decisions while avoiding the possibility of harming a real patient. Case studies can "foster critical thinking, collaboration, and competence" (Purtee et al., 2005, p. 307).

Day (2011) described the unfolding case study as similar to the typical case study. It is unique in its ability to focus on certain concepts that align to the learning objectives in a stepwise approach. In her discussion of the subject-centered classroom, she has described the unfolding case study as a central learning strategy that the students and nurse educator work through together as a team. As the case study unfolds, the educator is able to providc just-in-time teaching to fill in knowledge gaps or deepen understanding of the students in the classroom. Day's description of how the educator and students work as a collaborative team to provide the best virtual care to the case study subject fits perfectly with the flipped classroom. The flipped classroom may be able to offer one additional advantage that allows for more intense, individual student engagement in the teaching strategy of the unfolding case study. As students work either individually or in smaller groups on such a case, they are required to be more invested in the care and progression of the case study patient. There are simply fewer students in these smaller groups to dominate the question-and-answer interchange that occurs between the faculty and students compared to the larger class setting.

Due to the application of nursing concepts and interventions inherent in the use of case studies, case-based learning is highly recommended for the in-class activities of the flipped classroom for nursing education. As one might imagine, the case scenario requires students to apply the content learned in the off-load assignments. Such a strategy fits both the application of higher-level learning objectives and the need for more active learning. The remaining question might be where to access the best patient case scenarios for in-class activities. There are many texts now available that are full of case studies for nursing and medical education. Some of the textbooks used for nursing education courses may also have a case study within the assigned chapter that can be used for the in-class learning. Additionally, computerized case studies have become a more technology-based option popular with the digital native generation. Although these are excellent resources, there is the possibility that these types of generic case studies do not match closely enough the learning objectives for the unit. Often the nurse educator desires that students learn about the care of a particular type of patient with specific issues. In these cases, the nurse educator is encouraged to create a case study of his or her own. Doing so does take a bit of additional time and effort. However once completed, the case can be used over and over, as well as revised and changed to meet the exact learning needs of the current time.

Developing an Effective and Challenging Case Study

Although there are many approaches to development of case studies, the best case studies come from a nurse educator's professional, clinical experiences. In order to fashion the case study to fit the desired student learning outcomes perfectly, nurse educators can use their own clinical experiences and make a few minor adjustments. Perhaps there is a need for a case scenario in which the nurse educator has no first-hand experience. In these cases, asking another faculty member or those whom the educator has worked with in the past to share a patient scenario from their clinical experiences can offer a valid case that fits the needs of the classroom. When case studies are developed from real-life experiences, they cannot help but be authentic. Everything, or almost everything, about the case scenario can fit an actual clinical experience because it was first a true clinical experience before its debut in the learning environment. It is difficult to argue that the best simulations of real nursing practice are those that actually occurred. The realistic history within make them the most valid and reliable kinds of scenarios from which to teach.

When developing a case study for students from professional clinical experiences, there are a few things to keep in mind. It should go without saying, but protection of past patients and their families with alias names and fictitious settings is absolutely necessary. Some cases are so bizarre that they may be able to be identified just by sharing parts of the case with the students. In these situations, consider whether it would be best to share only the diagnosis and a few other details. Particularly if the scenario occurred in a rural setting or one with a smaller population, the chances of inadvertently revealing the true identity of either the patient or the family are understandably much higher. Most likely seasoned nurse educators understand the importance of protecting the patient and family identity to their utmost ability.

After reviewing the learning objectives for the unit, the nurse educator should extract the specific student outcomes that are desired with use of the case study. If the diagnosis or formation of a differential diagnosis for a certain condition is within the objectives, the case study should lead the student to answer questions about their development. If one of the main goals of the unit and case study would be for the student(s) to recognize the patient who is experiencing an anaphylactic reaction, the case study should lead students from the history through to the signs and symptoms of anaphylaxis, asking them to identify in the case certain key aspects of recognizing this condition in their patient. Think ahead of time about the four or five key learning points that students must learn in order to successfully complete the unit. Then weave these key learning points into the case scenario at hand.

Case studies can be used in different ways within the classroom setting. Shorter case studies may only take 30 minutes or an hour of class time for students to complete. Others may take all semester to complete as they unfold gradually throughout the semester and address many learning objectives in the process. I often use what I call the "two-part case study." This case study has two main progressions of patient care that are both completed within the live class time and match the learning objectives for the unit. The students split into groups where they work to answer the questions about the first part of the case study. The entire class comes together for a discussion about their answers to questions in part one of the case study. Great discussion can develop around different care choices by different groups including rationale. After a short break, students come back to the classroom and dive into the second part of the case study.

For the nurse practitioner students, the second part of a two-part case study often focuses on a return visit of the patient the students took care of in part one case study office visit. Students have mentioned that they find this approach very helpful. They are allowed to think through patient care in an evolution, much like the actual primary care clinical settings they are in the same semester. For undergraduate student nurses, the case progression might include day one of care for the first part of the case study followed by day two. Day two could also be focused on the discharge of the patient from the hospital setting.

Think of the possibilities for such a case study with the associated patient teaching, clinical responsibilities, holistic care considerations, and group charting. The idea of collective charting came about by watching students in the clinical setting help each other with their charting skills. Collective charting in a student group can be quite helpful, because some students have strength in this area and teach others their charting abilities while completing the case study. Ending a case study with some sort of charting is highly recommended. Requiring this step of documentation within a case study not only allows the students to practice this very important skill, but also reminds them that their care is not complete until their charting is finished.

An additional way to use the two-part case study involves the use of two separate and unrelated two-step case studies assigned to two different groups of students. There is a risk of confusing the reader when trying to explain this particular strategy, but the idea is good enough to take that risk! Imagine a group of 36 students split into 6 groups containing 6 students each. Three of the groups of 6 students begin on patient case study "A" while the others begin to work on patient case study "B." For the first part of class, the students answer part one of their assigned two-part case study. Instead of a discussion with the entire class, the last part of the assigned case study for all groups is to create a patient hand-off note for the next shift. The hand-off note the students developed for case study "A" is given to the student groups who were assigned case study "B" and vice versa. After the break, the students who originally were working on case study "A" pick up care for case study "B" beginning with part two of the two-part case study. They do not have additional details of what the students did for the patient in the case study other than what was written in the hand-off note. Students who originally were assigned case study "B" start taking care of case study "A" for the second part of the two-part case study. After both parts of the case study are completed, all students come back to the larger class group to discuss both cases together. The hand-off notes from group to group become a point of discussion. The importance of writing a strong hand-off note for the next shift of nurses comes to light.

One may also assign students to create case studies themselves for use within the larger classroom. This can be an individual assignment or one that is done within a small group. Having students create a case study requires them to understand much of the pathophysiology, nursing care, and medication management of the conditions they are learning about in any particular nursing course. This can be a successful approach, but by and large student-developed case studies are not very challenging. Perhaps this is a good place to start for the novice student. In this case, the nurse educator can embellish the case study to increase its complexity as the discussion about the case ensues in the class or within small group settings. For example, if the student-written case study asks for the top three signs of hypothyroidism, the nurse educator could add a question about why these signs manifest within the body. The nursing care or interventions associated with each of the three signs of a condition could also be an add-on question to increase the critical thinking and complexity of a more simple or straightforward case study.

An example of a case study focused on gestational diabetes developed for the advanced practice registered nursing (APRN) students can be found in **Table 7-2**. This example shows the development of desired student learning outcomes, actual case presentation, and questions within the case study developed to target the desired learning outcomes. The discussion and direction that occurs during such a case study within the classroom is hard to describe. Each time the case studies are used, they tend to bring up different questions and paths of learning depending on what types of questions the students ask. The instructor may ask different questions on the spot verbally that are not necessarily a part of the written case study to target additional learning outcomes that arise during the process of the case study. The end result resembles some of the discussions about patient care one may be able to recall from his or her own experiences on the nursing floor or in the primary clinical area. Discussing different ideas of a patient scenario with colleagues to arrive at the destination of the most excellent patient care occurs on a regular basis and mirrors this case study atmosphere seen in the classroom.

Table 7-2 Development of a Case Study Using Clinical Experience

Key Desired Learning Outcomes	Case Study Patient Scenario (abridged)	Case Study Questions
Part 1 – Diagnostic Ability		
1. Diagnosis of gestational diabetes mellitus (GDM) in primary care obstetrics setting. 2. Knowledge of when to test for GDM in prenatal care. 3. Knowledge of what blood testing to order for GDM. 4. Identification of risk factors for GDM.	39-year-old Caucasian female G3 P1, 2001. Ht = 5ft 6in – Wt =166, 24 3/7 weeks gestation, no problems. Total weight gain 10# <u>Urine</u> – Neg glucose, Neg protein, Neg Leuks <u>First child</u> 7.5# boy, no complications, SVD without instrumentation. <u>Second pregnancy</u> SVD, 5# boy, postdates by 2 weeks, complicated with fetal diagnosis of trisomy 18, live birth but child passed away at 4 months of age. Pt refused to complete GDM testing in second pregnancy due to trisomy diagnosis. <u>Third pregnancy</u> occurred at age 38, 1 month after 2nd boy passed away. <u>Family Hx</u> – Father type 2 DM, COPD, Obesity, HTN Mother – HTN, anxiety/depression	1. Mrs. X is here to visit you in the clinic today. She has had prenatal care since week 10 of this pregnancy. Discuss with your group members what you as the FNP will be doing for her prenatal visit today—please write your answer in the space below: 2. Does Mrs. X have any risk factors for gestational diabetes? If so, what and why? 3. Mrs. X asks if she will need any additional testing today and when she should come back to the clinic. Please educate her using the space below:

(*Continues*)

Table 7-2 Development of a Case Study Using Clinical Experience (Continued)

Key Desired Learning Outcomes	Case Study Patient Scenario (abridged)	Case Study Questions
Part 2 – APN Care of GDM Patient		
1. Communication of testing showing GDM is positive with patient/family. 2. Ordering glucose monitoring for GDM patient. 3. Referral practices within primary care for GDM patient. 4. Reading blood glucose records to determine patient control of GDM. 5. Discussion of follow-up care necessary for GDM patient. 6. Common complications of GDM pregnancy for baby.		4. Mrs. X's 1 hour GTT results are in your inbox within the EMR and reads 150mg/dl, what is your next action? 5. Also within your inbox is a phone message from Mrs. X who is calling for her blood tests. You call her back—in the space below, develop the conversation as you would expect it to transpire with Mrs. X: 6. What is your next action with Mrs. X? In order to not give away the answers, the nurse educator can give some additional clues about testing with the just-in-time teaching technique. For example, when the students say they would order a 3 hour GTT, the nurse educator then puts on the board or computer screen/projector the results of this test and asks the group to again make a care decision and a phone call. The next section can be dictated verbally to have the students consider referral services they will order. Additionally, a fictitious home blood glucose monitoring record is provided to each group to analyze. According to whether the patient is in good or poor glucose control, next treatment decisions are made as a group.

If the course concepts and learning objectives are focused on learning the care and diagnosis (advanced practice) of gestational diabetes mellitus (GDM) in primary care, educators should write down the key aspects they wish students to learn. For this example, these may include: (1) When to order tests for GDM detection; (2) Identification of risk factors for GDM; (3) Detection of clinical signs and symptoms of GDM.

Case-based teaching is a strategy that requires nursing students to apply their knowledge of off-load materials within the in-class setting in a very meaningful and realistic manner. Use of case studies during the in-class period of the flipped classroom is a favorite of flipping nurse educators for these reasons. The ability to teach in a type of virtual clinical environment cannot be underestimated. Before students initiate a nursing care action, they must first conceptualize that action, its rationale, and its most probable outcomes in a cognitive manner. Exercising this cognitive practice with realistic case studies while nursing faculty are there to help students correct errors in thinking and develop solid critical thinking in patient care scenarios holds a great deal of learning potential for nursing education.

Problem-Based Learning

Problem-based learning (PBL) is a pedagogical strategy that presents a problem to students that they must solve. In the process of solving the problem, learning occurs. In the traditional learning model, students are told what they need to know and then asked to apply it to a problem that they might encounter. Case studies are a great example of this traditional way to teach nurses how to care for patients and families. So how is PBL different than a case study? Well, PBL begins with presentation of a patient problem. The student must engage critical thinking and analysis skills to gather information about the problem and why it may be occurring before they can solve the problem. These steps in the PBL process lead students to learn what they need to know in order to solve the problem at hand.

Billings and Halstead (2005) list several advantages of using a PBL approach, including its ability to foster critical thinking, clinical reasoning, and active learning. An additional advantage might be PBL's reflection of what occurs day to day in nursing practice (both graduate and undergraduate). The practicing nurse is often faced with a patient problem to solve, and does not have the advantage of knowing all the facts necessary to solve the problem at hand. Teaching students to engage their investigative character and critical thinking ability to develop knowledge in order to solve patient problems sets them in a unique learning environment. Patients are rarely able to verbally tell the nurse what the problem is. Instead, they give the nurse clues and evidence through both subjective and objective means that need to be pieced together for a picture to emerge. Once the nurse is able to put those pieces together, they are able to move forward and solve the problem.

In a meta-analysis on the effect of PBL in nursing education, Shin and Kim (2013) analyzed 22 quantitative research-based articles between 1972 and 2012 with an experimental, quasi-experimental, descriptive comparative design. Analysis indicated that PBL offers many benefits to nursing education compared to traditional methods (use of lecture). Some of the benefits listed were greater student control over individual learning, positive student attitudes toward the method, and higher student satisfaction with PBL over traditional methods. The authors admitted that actual learning within PBL is difficult to accurately determine with the outcome measures used by most of the studies that had been reviewed. Overall, the authors felt the meta-analysis of PBL literature revealed a positive effect of the method on clinical education, student satisfaction, and psychomotor factors in the outcome domain within nursing education.

In the United Kingdom, Cooper and Carver (2012) developed a study to explore the experience of two cohorts of students within a mental health nursing course. Their qualitative study used focus groups of 6 to 8 students (n = 30 total) at the first week, mid-term, and the final week of the course about their experience with PBL in the course. Three main themes were identified from analysis of the focus group transcripts: moves to autonomy, surviving the groups, and the impact of PBL. Within the theme of "moves to autonomy," students voiced concerns about not knowing enough to solve the problems presented. Some felt that the method mimicked what would happen in the practice setting, and were positive about the guidance from faculty within this virtual experience. Participants felt that specific guidance from faculty was necessary for their successful learning in PBL. Students also preferred facilitators that would encourage them to question material and provide constructive criticism on the content and style of their work. Finally, participants voiced a desire to learn from the faculty who had experience in clinical nursing settings.

The theme of "surviving the groups" described student experiences of group work and the inherent interpersonal tensions that can occur within a group. Students did see small group work as attractive for the added mutual peer support and opportunity to share knowledge with one another. Student participants in this study had anxieties about their lack of experience with mental health issues, not being taken seriously by their peers, that the group work would not be effective, and the necessary reliance on other group members. Mid-term, the student participants felt that the success of PBL was largely dependent upon group cohesion and motivation of individual students. In the final focus groups, students shared their experience of building the unified group that performed at the expected level. They admitted that there was a process to learning how to work together and get used to the different personalities. After time, the students were able to work as a team rather than being forced into a group. As a result, they felt more comfortable challenging one another's ideas and quality of work in a professional manner (Cooper & Carver, 2012).

The final theme of the qualitative analysis was "impact of PBL." At the beginning of the course, student participants were hopeful that PBL would be an effective method of learning. By the end of the course, those hopes had been realized and students felt they were learning within the pedagogy. These students did express some negative effects of PBL including the necessity to work together with others, the fear that the depth of knowledge gained did not match their expectations, and the requirement of the student to be actively engaged in their learning. One participant stated (paraphrase) that PBL becomes what you want it to become (Cooper & Carver, 2012, p. 180). A particularly poignant quote from a participant highlights PBL in comparison to traditional lecture-based learning, "I don't like lectures...you only ever learn what the lecturer thinks is important" (Cooper & Carver, 2012, p. 179). This participant quote speaks volumes and originates from a student in the audience of nursing education.

PBL Activities

My favorite PBL activity for the in-class session is called "Expert of the Day." When the content to be taught focuses primarily around problems that will be encountered in patient populations, this is a great teaching strategy. For the off-load assignment, each member of a student group is assigned to become the "resident expert" for a particular topic. When teaching high-risk obstetrical topics, each student is assigned a topic. For example, assume that one student is assigned to be the expert on preterm labor. The student must read additional articles about preterm labor, watch a specific video, and come to class prepared to answer the other students' questions about preterm labor. When the PBL scenarios are distributed, the student who is the resident expert in preterm labor is "consulted" by the rest of the group to help them solve the problem that has been assigned.

The peer teaching that occurs during this process is nothing short of phenomenal. There is a fear that the resident expert will be no sort of expert at all, ignoring the assignment to become the expert prior to coming to class. This is not the case at all. It seems that when students are given the chance to really focus on one topic and be the expert for the rest of the group or class, they take great pride and are incredibly responsible with this task. When the strategy was introduced to the students, they were immediately worried that they would only learn about the topic that they were assigned. For example, if they were the resident expert in preterm labor, then they would not be prepared to answer exam questions about other topics such as pre-eclampsia. Instead, they discovered that their peers were so knowledgeable, that they learned all they needed to know through that peer instruction. All students were encouraged to read through shorter assignments related to all topics to increase their understanding. However, students shared their surprise in the amount of learning that occurred in the peer-to-peer teaching process.

The PBL strategy of expert of the day does require a fair amount of just-in-time teaching and/or use of the mini lecture. Students tend to get stuck in the PBL process in about the same places. Using a mini-lecture provides the faculty member with a great stopping point to pull everyone back together for a quick discussion and explanation session. In the spirit of PBL, it is okay to make the students attempt to answer the questions by themselves rather than providing an answer as the faculty expert. After all, discovering knowledge to solve the problem is part of the PBL process of learning. When students have questions during this pedagogy, ask them to begin working through the problem verbally together within their group. The educator can be there to guide them and give them small clues, but having them figure things out on their own contributes to that deeper learning experience and self-discovery that are connected to the development of critical thinking.

An additional PBL strategy for the advanced practice nursing students is called "on-call day." This strategy was developed on my first job as an APRN in which I was required to take call for obstetrical and gynecology patients without any formal training. Particularly with a high-stakes obstetrical population, making treatment decisions over the phone is a complicated skill requiring strong critical thinking skills. Putting students in this type of virtual call environment forces them to make critical decisions about patient care in a short amount of time. The strategy could be altered and used with undergraduate students as well, but registered nurses (RN) do not typically have to take calls from patients in their RN roles. Taking calls is often an expected role of an APRN, but a skill that is not often taught in APRN programs.

The off-load assignment for the on-call day includes reading and short videos to teach basic signs and symptoms as well as danger signs for common conditions that patients use the on-call system for on a regular basis. I've used this strategy for the unit on common obstetrical problems. These problems could be a result of normal pregnancy processes, or more serious conditions in need of more emergent treatment. Students must consider the signs and symptoms that each patient calls in with to arrive at their ultimate care decision to treat at home or send the patient in for further evaluation. Instead of breaking into groups, students work together with the faculty to answer "calls" that come in from different patients with various problems. Students must practice real-time PBL as the nursing faculty takes the role of the patient who is calling with a problem for the students in the classroom to solve. Students must also decide what the best and most safe course of action would be for each scenario. For each treatment decision, students must include their rationale in the discussion.

Problem-based learning is a challenge for some nursing educators who have been in a certain educational paradigm for years and years. For these educators (this author included), *not* providing students with a quick answer but requiring them to find it on their own is a big educational challenge. Isn't that what the nursing educators are there for—to answer the students' questions? The answer is yes and no. It can take a while for some educators to understand that teaching is not about faculty members showing the students their vast knowledge and ability. Teaching nursing is about fostering knowledge and ability *within the student*. For some educators, it may be time to consider stepping back from the "show and tell" expert role in favor of a more supporting role. Doing so has the potential to foster student development and learning within a safe environment. Within the realm of PBL, the educator must assume a more passive role and allow students to think through patient problems on their own. Struggling with difficult questions to find the best answer is part of what nurses do every day. Giving students all the answers in the PBL model will actually stunt the critical thinking process and inhibit student learning that could have occurred naturally. Not left to learn on their own, but guided in the right direction, students can be quite successful in maneuvering difficult patient problems.

Role Play and Student Acting

Role play is described by Billings and Halstead as "a dramatic approach in which individual assume the roles of others" (2005, p. 305). Role play is typically used by educators when teaching students about communication with others. Most of the time, the communication is between the student and their future patient. Other times, it is communication between other members of the healthcare team. Billings and Halstead describe role play as a usually unscripted and spontaneous verbal interchange that is observed and analyzed by a third party. The third party observing and critiquing the interaction is usually the nurse educator, but could also be student peer.

When using role play, Billings and Halstead (2005) have recommended that educators plan with three main stages in mind. The first is *briefing*, where the stage is set and explanation of the objectives of the exercise are reviewed with the students. Second is the *running*, or acting out of the role play. Third in the sequence is a *debriefing* session including a discussion, analysis, and evaluation of the running session of the role play learning activity. This third step is the most valuable in terms of student learning about interactions and reactions of the role play. The ability to dissect the role play and identify positive and negative aspects of an interaction allows students to reflect on their therapeutic communication ability. Within this debriefing session, students learn about effective and ineffective communication techniques, body language, and cultural aspects of communication in a reflective manner.

Advantages of role play include the ability for students to observe themselves and get a bird's eye view of themselves in action. They become more aware of how their verbal and nonverbal actions can steer a conversation with a patient or family member. Billings and Halstead (2005) include these additional advantages of increasing student observational skills, decision-making skills, comprehension of complex human behaviors, and connection to real-life scenarios the students will encounter in clinical settings. As students view their interactions and those of their peers, they are able to have immediate feedback about their skills and actions. There is virtually no cost in the use of role play and very little preparation in terms of handouts because role play typically uses spontaneous interactions between student groups or pairs.

Role play also has some disadvantages, which may keep educators from using the strategy. Reluctance of students to participate and fully invest in role play may be the largest barrier. Some students tend to be more theatrical and really engage in the process, making role play a very valuable experience for student learning. Other students despise the idea of having to "play" someone they are not. The additional feedback from students includes their discomfort being under the observational microscope as they interact with a peer during role play. Students have a valid point that they interact differently while observed or when being videotaped than they would in a live situation with a patient. As Billings and Halstead (2005) warn, role play can be a costly use of class time if not planned appropriately.

Hubbard (2014) has successfully used role play in the development of psychiatric mental health nurse practitioner student competencies. As the author stated, students may be extremely proficient with testing and written assignments, but lack proficiency in application of clinical skills. Customized role play was used as a strategy for student-centered learning and its ability for students to conceptualize a case that integrated cultural, social, and patient interaction concepts integral to the advance practice psychiatric role. Hubbard also used the pedagogy due to its ability to engage students on the cognitive, affective, and psychomotor domains of learning. When used as a teaching strategy, the author recommended concurrently running role-play pairs with the instructor circulating, correcting, and assisting as needed. When used for testing or evaluation of student competency, the faculty role was defined as observation and evaluation without any feedback given until the culmination of the interaction. Whether used as a teaching strategy or for evaluation of competency, a debriefing period was always used as the final step of the role-play process. Seen as an opportunity for students to close learning gaps and achieve entry-level proficiency of advanced practice nursing, Hubbard recommends the use of well-developed, customized role play to provide rich, student-centered learning experiences.

Similarly, Krimshtein et al. (2011) implemented training for intensive care unit (ICU) nurses within five veterans hospitals focused on interdisciplinary communication with families in which role play was used as a primary strategy. Postprogram self-evaluation scores improved significantly, with nurses feeling that the case scenarios and role play were a very effective way to practice and receive feedback about their communication abilities. All participants reported that they would recommend a similar program of training to their colleagues. Additional affirmation of the use of role play in this program included participants' feeling of increased self-awareness of their role in the interdisciplinary team and a higher level of confidence voicing their opinions about patient care and participation in family meetings. The authors recommended role play as an effective teaching and learning strategy for its student-centered focus and ability to allow practice of real-life situations.

Role play in the flipped classroom can take on another twist in the form of students playing or acting out scenarios not directly related to therapeutic communication. Caputi and Englemann (2005) have discussed an example of using role play in a unique way to display the actions of diabetes as shared by Dr. Marie Colucci from a community college in California. To explain the physiology and pathophysiology of diabetes to students, several student volunteers are asked to come to the front of the class to play the cell, insulin, and sugar roles. The cell players hook arms to make a circle as Dr. Colucci explains to the class the physiology of normal cell metabolism. The students playing the role of insulin then hook up with the sugar and together then enter the circle of the cell students and provide energy. Although not listed as a part of the role play described, the cell students could be inactive, standing still until the insulin and sugar enter the ring. After the sugar/insulin enters the cell student ring, the students could become "active" and move slowly around in a circle to simulate addition of energy to the cell, which leads to the ability to move. Then the group can act out what happens with the pathophysiology of Type 1 and Type 2 diabetes with the help of the faculty member. An additional step would be to show students how medications, exercise, stress, illness, and other factors may affect diabetes in the patient's body.

I have used student acting in a similar way as an active learning strategy for an undergraduate obstetrics course. Learning a unit focused on newborn care, students were split into groups and assigned the role of a newborn with a condition. The goal of the group was to convince the nursery nurse (the faculty member) why they were the most important baby in the nursery in need of attention over the other babies. The groups included hypoglycemia, ABO incompatibility, pathologic jaundice, cold stress, transient tachypnea of the newborn, and hypothermia. More conditions could be added if desired. Students were given time during class to come up with the most convincing argument with some specific guidelines. The guidelines asked students to cover a brief definition of the condition, risk factors, signs and symptoms of the condition, necessary physical assessments, and an argument of why they were the most important baby in the nursery in need of the nurse's attention. After students presented their cases, the students took time to reflect on each diagnosis and presentation individually. Students were extremely creative in their presentations of their assigned baby diagnosis adding to student ability to remember key parts of each diagnosis for later application and testing. Students were very positive about the experience and asked for additional similar strategies for future classes. The ideas for this type of acting are endless.

Debate

Debate as an active teaching and learning strategy has been used for years within all types of learning environments. The ability to debate, to take a particular stance on a subject, requires a student to engage in a deep level of learning in order to be successful. The critical thinking that is involved in the preparation for a debate offers an effective application learning approach for the in-class session of the flipped classroom. Not only do the students have to prepare to defend their topic with a substantive statement of support, but they also need to use forethought in anticipation of questions from their peers that will rebuke that statement of support. Therefore, preparation for rebuttal comments can involve a great deal of investigative action and abstract understanding of a particular topic as well.

Billings and Halstead (2005) described debate as a process of inquiry on a proposition aimed at demonstrating either the falsehood or truth of a subject. It involves the development of logical, ordered argument used in an oral defense. The recognition of evidence to support or refute a certain topic should be an essential component of debate when used in the nursing education classroom. Students must use both inductive and deductive reasoning skills. Cultivation of their ability to identify relationships between and among the debated subjects, evidence, popular opinion, and cultural expectation are additional learning benefits of the strategy. Billings and Halstead recommended use of this strategy in coursework that requires higher-level cognitive thinking of nursing students.

In the flipped classroom model, assignment of a debate side or position could be assigned for off-load learning. Reminding students that rebuttal is a necessary part of any debate will navigate off-load learning of both their assigned position and that of the opposing position as well. Debates are best used with a consistent format that should be shared with the students ahead of time. For example, the debate may begin with an opening comment session in which students share the substantive support statement of their position including associated evidence. Time limitations should be set for each part of the debate and held firm. After opening statements from each side, presentation of affirming and negating viewpoints are shared, followed by any rebuttal comments. The debate culminates in a summary period from each side. Some educators using debate as a teaching strategy have students spend a moment of reflection about the debate. This period of reflection is focused on an attempt to objectively think about which side essentially "won" the debate by bringing forth evidence-based support rather than only public or popular opinion. A discussion of evidence-based practice often naturally follows.

One limiting factor of using debate in the flipped classroom may be the size of the debating groups. Billings and Halstead recommended groups of five students with two students debating for a topic, two students debating against the topic, and one student taking the role of moderator. Considering student numbers in a nursing classroom can be in excess of 30, the feasibility of using debate while engaging each student in active learning is in question. Of course, several debates could take place simultaneously within the classroom. This approach could bring a loud, unmanageable activity full of chaos. It is still possible for learning to occur in such an environment, but the ability for faculty to control, moderate, and teach in such an environment may be substantially stunted. In a larger class, the debate could go on with the majority of students in the audience, gauging the effectiveness of the debating students. Learning can still occur in this process, but taking so many students out of the active learning role in this scenario pulls into question the interactivity of the method. For these reasons, debate may be more effectively used with smaller groups of students to promote truly active learning of each student within the classroom at the highest level possible.

Concept or Mind Mapping

Mind mapping or concept mapping is a teaching and learning strategy that employs individual student learning of a phenomenon or concept with the use of visual imagery in a graphic display. Novak and Canas define concept maps as "graphical tools for organizing and representing knowledge" (2008, p. 1). The concept map represents how a particular student envisions concepts and how they are connected. Therefore, each student will develop his or her own unique concept map according to how the student has structured ideas and connections about concepts within the student's own cognitive atmosphere. Concept maps are individual student learning and expression of comprehension at its finest. Asking students to develop a concept map requires them to reflect on how their brain is linking concepts together.

Students may not be linking concepts together in their brain at all. Here is where the concept map as a teaching strategy is very useful. Making students think and learn about how concepts are related forces them into an abstract, three-dimensional view of patient care. The act of putting their thoughts on paper helps students connect their thoughts about concepts together with their readings, available evidence, nursing interventions, and patient care outcomes. Nursing students are attempting to pull past knowledge of pathophysiology, anatomy and physiology, and pharmacology together with current learning objectives to develop appropriate nursing interventions. The concept map provides a great strategy for students to pull past learning together with new concepts. In the realm of cognitive load theory, concept maps are a visual way to use a schema. The schema, if you will recall, is a previously known concept that is used by the brain to "scaffold" new information in a structured way. Students can use the visual vehicle of the concept map to show faculty (and themselves) how they understand the many-layered concepts and interventions necessary to carry out nursing care of patient conditions.

Orique and McCarthy (2015) examined the relationship between critical thinking and the use of concept maps and PBL together as a teaching strategy for undergraduate nursing students. Using a pretest, posttest quasi-experimental design, 49 student participants' care plans were assessed by researchers using the Holistic Critical Thinking Scoring Rubric (Cronbach's alpha of 0.88 was found with a pilot group prior to the study). Students in the course developed a care plan with typical teaching methods first, then were exposed to the intervention of concept mapping to develop additional care plans. Instruction on what a concept map was as well as an example was provided for student understanding. During this same time period, PBL was introduced as the primary instructional method. On the posttest evaluation, critical thinking scores were statistically significantly higher for the PBL, concept mapping session. Researchers noticed that before the PBL and concept mapping approach, students had difficulty communicating with clinical instructors about the nursing process and disease processes. Clinical instructors noted a decrease in this difficulty after use of the concept mapping, as well as demonstrated greater clinical reasoning and decision-making skills related to planning and implementing care for their patients. These findings coupled with reports from students that they felt more competent with the use of concept mapping make it a very valid teaching and learning method for nursing education.

Concept mapping used in conjunction with high-fidelity simulation has also proven to be a successful approach to the complex learning necessary in the nursing care of patients. Using an exploratory, correlational study, Samawi, Miller, and Haras (2014) used three National League for Nursing tools to measure the effects of simulation coupled with concept mapping on student self-confidence. Six different focus groups with student participants focused on how concept mapping influenced self-confidence in pediatric assessment and care. Three themes emerged including advanced assessment skills, increased critical thinking, and greater self-confidence. Although most of the positive outcomes of this study may be attributed to the use of high-fidelity simulation, exemplars of student concept maps were thought by researchers to demonstrate student ability to critically analyze pediatric simulation scenarios that could be applied to the practice setting.

In the world of medical education, Bixler, Brown, Way, Ledford, and Mahan (2015) used concept mapping with their fourth year medical students. Their nonexperimental pilot study used a pretest–posttest single group design to find if small group concept mapping would improve critical thinking. Critical thinking skills were measured using the California Critical Thinking Skill Test, a multiple-choice format involving seven subscales measuring aspects of critical thinking.

In terms of knowledge acquisition, when compared to pretest scores (average of 35%), posttest scores (50%, $p = <.001$) were significantly higher. The critical thinking scores were not significantly different between groups (pretest = 83.9 and posttest = 85.6). Although there was an improvement in the score, statistical significance was not able to be demonstrated. As stated by the researchers, scores were high on the pretest for these medical students. Therefore, additional increase in critical thinking due to the intervention might not have been able to be adequately measured. The end result found by the researchers was that concept mapping in conjunction with readings did improve content knowledge. Critical thinking ability of this medical student sample were initially high and did increase, but not at a statistically significant level.

Concept maps (in my humble opinion) are best done individually by students. Often used as an off-load assignment, the students can create a concept map of their understanding and either turn it in to the faculty member or present it to the class during the in-class session. Concept maps can also be completed in a small group. As a small group project, several brains and abstract ideas must come together to form one concept map representative of every member of a student group. Often used in conjunction with the jigsaw teaching strategy (see following section), concept maps developed by groups can be used to teach material in a peer instruction format. Hicks-Moore (2005) believes that small group concept map development is an effective teaching and learning tool that can bridge the gap between theory and practice. Kinchin and Hay (2005) used concept mapping in the classroom with student triads and found that differing knowledge structures of student participants equated to better student outcomes. Group brainstorming can also allow for sharing of ideas and new ways to envision concepts that may enhance understanding from one student to the next.

However used in the nursing classroom, concept mapping as a strategy should include clear guidance for students about what the concept map should include. Allowing creativity and individuality of how the concept map itself is created a must. If too strictly dictated by faculty in terms of conformity, the main theory behind development of the concept map for learning is ignored. Allow students to create on paper what their minds are perceiving. Doing so allows for the crux of student learning and understanding inherent in the strategy of concept mapping.

Jigsaw Teaching Strategy

The jigsaw teaching strategy was developed by Elliot Aronson, currently Professor Emeritus at the University of California (Jigsaw.org, 2015). The strategy was first used in his 1971 graduate classroom partly to diffuse racial tensions and inter-group hostility within Austin, Texas city school systems. In an attempt to shift the attention from the instructor to the students and engage every student in the class regardless of cultural aspects, language challenges, and knowledge levels led to development of the jigsaw method. Changing the class structure into smaller groups working together, each student was required to understand the content, as it was necessary, for them to teach it to one another (Jigsaw.org). By definition, the *jigsaw learning strategy* is a cooperative learning technique in which each student becomes a part of the larger learning atmosphere, much like smaller pieces of a larger puzzle. When each student's part in the learning is essential, each student becomes essential to the learning process as well.

The jigsaw has been used successfully in many nursing education classrooms, although it has not been empirically tested. Charania, Kauser, and Cassum (2001) discussed jigsaw as an effective cooperative learning experience for nursing students assisting in the development of critical thinking. Similar description and positive discussion about the method has been listed in earlier nursing publications (Ulrich & Glendon, 1995), and the technique has been presented at many nurse education conferences.

Wong and Driscoll (2007) used jigsaw learning with their physical therapy students, with student performance on quizzes being significantly higher than when independent study approach was used. Students in the study commented that the jigsaw helped them integrate prior coursework and apply knowledge together with student peers to solve complex patient cases. Students also felt a sense of individual responsibility to their group members due to the requirement to peer instruct. Comments from students indicated that the jigsaw allowed reflective and more expanded thinking abilities. The jigsaw has also been used in medical education, with a specific focus on prescribing skills with very positive results (Sim et al., 2014).

The jigsaw learning website (Jigsaw.org, 2015) explains how to use the jigsaw in 10 steps. In the nursing education classroom, a few very minor adjustments are recommended to decrease confusion among students and faculty. First, the class is divided into smaller groups of 5 to 6 students each. Each group is given a subject that matches the learning objectives for the day. The number of subjects must match the number of groups. In addition, the number of students in each group must match the number of subjects assigned. In a scenario where 6 subjects are assigned, then 6 groups of 6 students each should be formed (see **Figure 7-5**).

Take, for example, the concepts of learning cardiac physical assessment with a group of 36 students. In the 6-subject example, group A may be assigned to prepare a concept map or teaching guide of some sort focused on cardiac assessment using auscultation points on the chest wall. Group B could be assigned to create their materials around the peripheral aspects of cardiac assessment. Group C could focus on assessment and recognition of systolic murmurs, and group D could focus on diastolic murmurs. Group E could be assigned additional cardiac testing, such as venous jugular distention and hepatic reflux. Finally, group F could focus on the assessment and physiology of additional cardiac sounds such as S3, S4, and split S2. The original groups are given class time to develop either a concept map or some other form of teaching material. After the group materials are completed, each student in the group is assigned a number from 1 to 6. For example, Group A will then have student 1A, 2A, 3A, 4A, 5A, and 6A. Then all of the number "1" students form a group, "2" students form a group and so on until 6 new groups are formed. Each of the new groups will have a student from each of the original groups (for example, the "1" group will have students 1A, 1B, 1C, 1D, 1E, and 1F).

After the formation of the new groups, peer teaching is completed using materials created by the original group. Within the new group, the student who was part of creating the material will teach the others in his/her group. Using the example above, the student who created the teaching materials in group 1 on cardiac auscultation

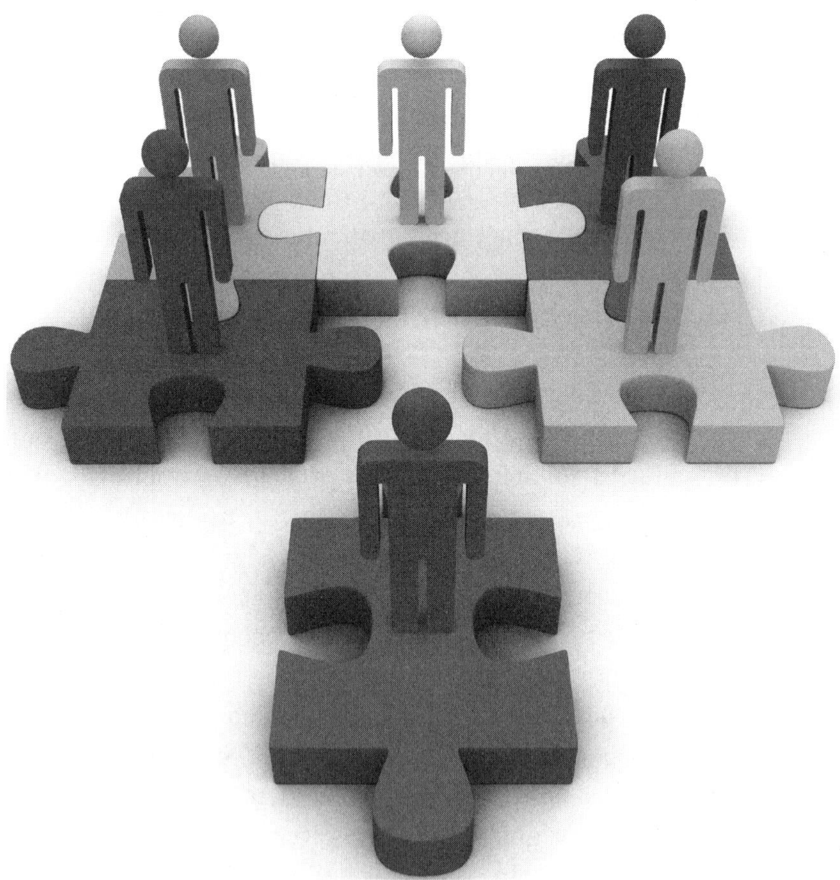

Figure 7-5 Jigsaw schematic.

assessment will teach the other students in their newly formed group. As the peer teaching takes place, the nursing instructor is available for questions and rotates with the groups to assist in correct instruction. Teaching times vary, but typically take around 10 to 15 minutes each. After all groups have rotated through each developed teaching material, the class is brought together in the larger group setting. Discussion of remaining questions can occur at this time, as well as just-in-time teaching focused on any areas of confusion. Some educators will also use a culmination assessment at this point, such as a clicker quiz, to solidify student understanding of the content.

Creating Algorithms

Similar to the concept mapping teaching strategy, students creating algorithms focused on nursing concepts and patient care is another in-class interactive strategy for use in the flipped classroom model. A bit more structured than a concept map, an algorithm is described as a step-by-step pictorial presentation of a procedure or process. Breaking steps of a clinical situation down into "yes" and "no" steps within an algorithm can assist student understanding of nursing intervention steps. Most effectively used with clinical scenarios, students are asked to create an algorithm that reflects the steps to be taken caring for a patient. If the learning objectives are directed toward learning care of the patient with hyperglycemia in the primary care setting, then students are asked to create an algorithm of this care process. Students can use their resources to make the algorithm evidence based. Algorithms can be created in small groups. Use of small groups is helpful due to the large amount of information and work necessary to create an accurate and evidence-based algorithm. An example of an algorithm is provided in **Figure 7-6**.

Quizzing

Quizzing students during the in-class time is a popular flipped classroom strategy for nursing education. Practice testing can help students solidify knowledge and exercise test-taking abilities.

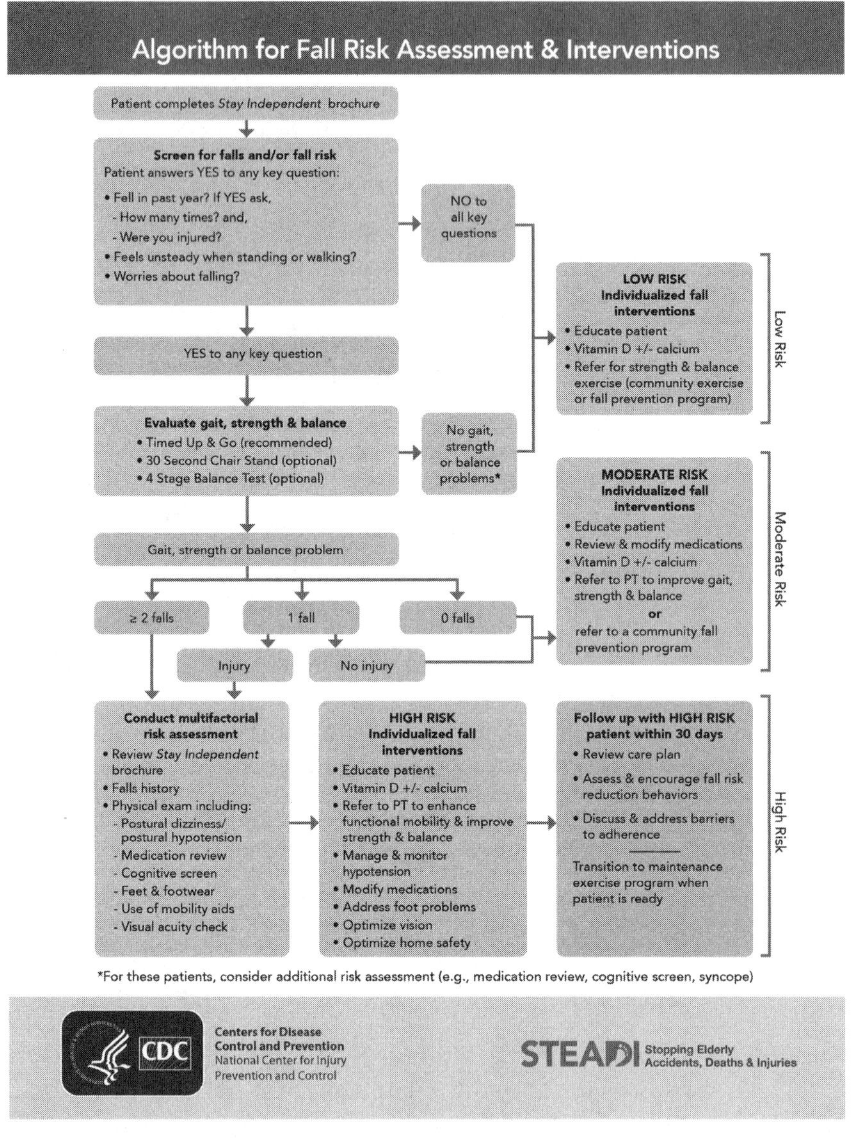

Figure 7-6 Algorithm example.
Courtesy of CDC

Butler and Roediger (2007) discovered that short-answer quizzing was the most effective form of testing to promote student retention of content. Repeated practice testing with feedback from instructors has also been shown to increase student confidence and performance during summative assessments (Butler, Karpicke, & Roediger, 2008).

In nursing, Cox-Davenport and Phelan (2015) investigated the use of adaptive (repetitive) quizzing with feedback to a level of mastery. A positive correlation was found between the use of adaptive testing and content mastery. These studies support the use of practice testing to improve student outcomes in a testing environment in higher education.

Practice testing can be delivered by paper and pencil or by means of a student response system. There are several student response systems to choose from. Some of these systems can even be run using student cell phones with text messaging. Many of the response software programs have instant percentages of correct and incorrect answers and instant grading that can be downloaded easily. There are also options for anonymous polling for sensitive subject matter. For example, during a unit focusing on drug and alcohol abuse, the instructor may want to poll the students in an anonymous manner to ask their experience with addictions of family members or friends.

Testing in groups or pairs for practice has the potential to enhance student learning of course material and testing process. Discussing the thought behind one's choice on a particular test question develops reasoning and analysis of test choices with a peer. Doing so can foster an environment of collaboration and open student thinking to a peer's reasoning. Use of testing as a teaching strategy is best done in a low-stakes environment. Allowing students to exercise their reasoning and explore their thought processes with other students and faculty can correct errors in thinking and increase student confidence levels.

Use of collaborative testing for summative assessments has been investigated in the literature. Gallagher (2009) studied the use of collaborative group testing as a strategy to promote active learning. It was found that collaborative testing did have a positive effect on student learning. Students felt that taking tests in a group helped them understand the content better and gave them a higher confidence level in their own knowledge. Students reported that they studied more with the group testing in order to be an effective member of the testing team. Exam grades in the student groups did not improve from previously used individual testing scores. Gallagher made an important point that much of the work nurses do in actual practice is accomplished while working with others. The group process and problem-solving atmosphere created by group testing can foster a culture of collaboration that emulates actual nursing practice in the process.

After using collaborative testing for several years, Duane and Satre (2014) have offered recommendations for implementation of the method for nursing faculty. It is their recommendation that students be randomly assigned to collaborative testing groups. Collaborative testing should be used for extra credit or minimal points to decrease the occurrence of grade inflation. Use of collaborative testing in high-stakes testing is not recommended. The faculty should assist students in application of critical thinking, collaboration, and problem solving skills during the collaborative testing process.

In my flipped classroom, I have used testing as a teaching strategy with positive results. Students are happy to be able to practice testing, and have commented that it does increase their confidence when taking the actual exams. Collaborative testing is a slippery slope, in my opinion. I have only used collaborative testing in practice mode and as a teaching strategy. One grade for several students on any exam does not allow for individual knowledge to be evaluated. Invariably, there is a student who really did know the correct answer, but was talked out of it or out voted by the other members of the testing group. Instead, I use what I call "consultation time" at the end of random exams. The students take the exam individually, but star two or three questions that they are not confident about. During the last 5 minutes (maximum) of the exam, students can consult with one other person (usually their thought partner). Students are free to keep their exam answers the same or change them after they consult. I am careful to warn that if I see any comparison of answers on every question rather than collaboration, they lose the collaboration time entirely. I only use this approach when I have a smaller group of students that I can closely monitor during the collaboration time. Students have spoken positively about the experience to collaborate on one or two questions without having to change their answers. Other than this method of collaboration on exams for an actual grade, I only use testing as a teaching strategy where no punitive action can result.

Gaming

Use of gaming as pedagogy, although fun, exciting, and engaging, does not require higher-ordered thinking from the students. Students are mostly faced with a short question and quick rote response or answer within such a pedagogical format. Gaming tends to only engage two or three students at a time and leaves the other students out of the learning loop (depending on the game). Nursing students are generally very competitive as well, setting up an atmosphere that can quickly get out of control and interfere with true learning within the classroom. For these reasons, it is recommended to reserve gaming for a quick review of the material at the beginning of the class rather than letting it be the focus of the in-class activities with students.

Closing the In-Class Session

Bringing the students back together as a group at the end of the in-class session is a great way to end the class. During this time, evaluation of student understanding can be assessed in either a formal or informal way. Some educators will have a brief discussion with the students in the class that is focused on the learning objectives for the day. One approach is to hand out a worksheet that includes the learning objectives for the unit with blank spaces underneath. Have the students write out how they achieved each learning objective. A short quiz either on paper or with a classroom response system can also help to solidify understanding and help students answer any remaining questions about the content. Some educators may simply engage students in an additional Q & A session to answer any questions about content or clear up student confusion.

Closing the class together as a group also allows the nurse educator to prepare students for the next in-class session. Discussion of off-load assignments, reminders about faculty expectations, and assistance for students in time management can be covered. Help students plan ahead, and ask them when they will complete off-load assignments for the upcoming class. Doing so will help students with time management skills and promote once again the expectation for completion of any off-load assignments before the next class period. Of course, the nurse educator must have any assignments, videos, and other off-load materials ready for students to access ahead of time. A typical time frame is one week prior to the in-class session. Ask the students to write down when they will be completing off-load materials during the upcoming week. Students setting aside time that is dedicated to the off-load assignments can help them plan for their upcoming week and take ownership of their own learning.

Challenges During In-Class Time

Managing In-Class Time

Managing the in-class time is best done with a well-thought-out plan. One of the biggest challenges associated with the in-class management is correctly estimating the time it will take for students to complete interactive learning activities. A time-management planning template is helpful to keep the class on track and use time in the most efficient manner (see **Figure 7-7**). The first time the class is flipped, use the template to keep track of the amount of time each in class activity took. Doing so can make future time estimations of similar in-class activities much more accurate the next time the class is flipped.

Time is fluid in the flipped classroom. Estimating time for in-class learning activities may change from one class of students to the next. For this reason, always plan for additional learning activities just in case the original plan did not take as much time as expected. A case study that took last semesters' students 30 minutes may take the current students an hour or more. Be prepared for these types of time fluctuations and don't be stressed or upset

Estimated Time	Activity	Actual Time
15 min 0800–0815	Q & A session	
10 min 8015–0825	Explanation of in-class activities, expectations for learning today	
35 min 0825–0900	Cardiac Care Case Study	
10 min 0900–0910	BREAK	
60 min 0910–1010	Group discussion of case study	
10 min 1010–1020	BREAK	
10 min 1020–1030	Closing Q & A	
20 min 1030–1050	Clicker quiz with discussion	

Figure 7-7 In-class time management.

if time estimated for activities does not match reality. Instead, be prepared with some additional activities to fill in unexpected time left over. Here are some ideas the nurse educator can keep in a back pocket for extra learning after the planned interactivities have been completed:

1. Keep several evidence-based articles about the topic at hand ready for students to read and report on to the rest of the class if there is extra time available.
2. Create a summary assessment, such as a quiz or worksheet, that solidifies and tests student knowledge about the content. Hand it out for students to complete and discuss if there is additional time to do so.

3. Have students begin a reflective journal about the topics learned and activities completed during the in-class time. When extra time is available, have students complete a journal entry about their experiences. Be sure to have specific journaling questions ready for the students to journal about. They often have a hard time coming up with things to write about and reflect upon by themselves.
4. Have a set of 3 X 5 index cards ready. If there is extra time, have each student write down three "take-home points" from the content learned that day. Have students share their take-home points keeping a tally on the whiteboard or computer.

The Not-So-Engaged Student

Many nurse educators share a common concern and question about the use of the flipped classroom. What if students come unprepared to class? The reality is that some students will come unprepared to class. This is an unavoidable fact in the world of adult education. It might be that this particular question is really masquerading as a more general bias against the flipped classroom and is not related to the flipped classroom at all. The first thought would be how educators have been able to determine if students were ready to come to a lecture-based class? Is it completely necessary to quiz the students and make sure they've completed their readings before any lecture can begin? There are certainly some educators that do quiz students over their readings before they begin lecture. But does quizzing students before lecture make them more prepared for lecture? Does it make them more interested in the content or the lecture itself? Perhaps taking a look at what student motivation for completing the assigned readings really is in the first place would be helpful.

One thing that I've learned after years of teaching is that I cannot control my students' activities outside of the classroom. I have had to give up the idea that every student will be 100% prepared for class every day I teach. It took me a long time to realize that educators cannot make students complete readings, watch videos, or be interested in the in-class activities. Students must be internally and externally motivated to learn. Adult learners need to decide for themselves what that motivation to learn the material is and how strong it is. Educators can certainly help motivate students in many ways by providing a quality pedagogical experience for students. Perhaps we can go back to a question asked earlier in the text focused on individual definitions of success. It would most likely be safe to say that the definition of success might be different for students than for educators. The best educators can do is share their expectations, be clear in their directions, and support student learning in the best way they can.

After discussing the flipped classroom with several nurse educators, preparation for in-class activities in the world of the nursing education flipped classroom is not as big of an issue as one might imagine. Nurse educators are blessed to teach professional-based content that their students really want to learn. Nursing will be each student's career. Most (close to all!) students really want to learn the content the nurse educator is teaching because they will be using it every day in their future nursing practice. It is true that nurse educators still run into that occasional student who is uninterested and not motivated. But wouldn't that student still be in the classroom if lecture was used? It would just be more difficult to pick that student out of the lecture audience. The in-class activities of the flipped classroom do not allow the unmotivated, disengaged student to hide in the crowd. If anything, this is another positive aspect of flipped learning. Faculty can identify these students and work with them to increase understanding and hopefully motivation to learn as well.

There are also students in the flipped classroom model that are just not engaged in the in-class activities. There are a number of ways to deal with this scenario. The way a nurse educator approaches the uninterested student depends on personality and educational style. After discussing the situation with other flipping nurse educators, most choose to have a discussion with the student who is not participating. Reinforcing faculty expectations with each student in a face-to-face meeting has been offered as an effective approach.

One faculty member puts in writing her expectations for participation in the class activities. The educator schedules a meeting with the student face to face to review the written expectations together. A copy of the written document is given to the student along with expectations of improvement for future in-class sessions. Some educators allot points to the students for class participation. However, these points are typically a small portion of the overall grade. Therefore, they do not make much of a dent in the student grade if taken away for lack of involvement. By and large, a discussion with the student is a logical first-step approach that has proven to be effective for many flipping educators.

It is also possible to have a student who just doesn't like the flipped classroom model. There are, of course, many reasons for this preference, some that the student will not be willing to divulge. The best advice to provide faculty is, *"It's okay!"* Some students don't like lecture, some students don't like videos, some students don't like group work, and some just don't like any approach that requires what is perceived as more work. It is a fact of life in the educational world. *We cannot please everyone, but we can teach everyone!* Try to remember that flipping the classroom increases student engagement and critical thinking. The educator is doing what is best for student learning, even though some students do not appreciate those efforts. At the end of the day, the student will have learned the content, and that is the important factor in the flipping equation.

Students Who Do Not Come to Class

Students who do not come to class is a very valid and important issue. It is completely understandable that there are some nursing educators very concerned about the flipped classroom taking educational time and quality away from nursing programs. Some authors writing about the flipped classroom in higher education within the current literature have admitted that their class attendance when flipping the classroom is less than an anecdotally higher attendance to their lecture-based courses. Perhaps the question is, "Are these educators using the flipped classroom appropriately?" The question of how students are adequately educated about the flipped classroom is in question. Are these educators appropriately using Bloom's taxonomy, specifically lower-level objectives for off-load within recorded or online lecture materials? When flipping is done correctly, the students will not be able to do well in a flipped course unless they attend the in class or face-to-face sessions. Within these face-to-face sessions, the students should be applying the information at a higher level of learning taxonomy rather than engaging in activities that produce a repetition of content.

Conclusion

In conclusion, the in-class portion of the flipped classroom is full of exciting learning and student engagement activities. The more faculty use the flipped model, the more creative and innovative the in-class activities tend to become. Starting with a solid plan including a template with time estimations can help keep the in-class sessions more structured and on track. Be certain to choose in-class activities that build upon the off-load assignments. Have students complete activities during the in-class session that require them to learn higher-ordered objectives. Be confident in the approach and use of the flipped classroom and do not apologize to students for using the method. Flipping educators are working harder to invest in their students' learning, and that is nothing to apologize about! Take the time to plan for any excess time left over during the in-class session and keep track of the timing of activities used. Have fun with the method and don't forget to evaluate your flipped classroom as well. Flipping can be a successful teaching and learning strategy. The in-class activities are really the star of the show in the whole process of flipped learning. Having time to work with students on a more individual basis can provide a deeper learning experience for students and a better understanding of student learning by nurse educators. The in-class activities are vital to engaging the students in the classroom. Be creative and step out with some new and innovative active learning ideas during the in-class time with students.

References

Austria, M. J., Baraki, K., & Doig, A. K. (2013). Collaborative learning using nursing student dyads in the clinical setting. *International Journal of Nursing Education Scholarship, 10*(1), 1–8.

Bermann, J., & Sams, A. (2012). *Flip your classroom: Reach every student in every class every day.* Eugene, OR: International Society for Technology in Education.

Billings, D. M., & Halstead, J. A. (2005). *Teaching in nursing: A guide for faculty.* St. Louis, MO: Elsevier Saunders.

Bixler, G. M., Brown, A., Way, D., Ledford, C., & Mahan, J. D. (2015). Collaborative concept mapping and critical thinking in fourth-year medical students. *Clinical Pediatrics, 54*(9), 833–839.

Butler, A. C., & Roediger, H. L. (2007). Testing improves long-term retention in a simulated classroom setting. *European Journal of Cognitive Psychology, 19*(4/5), 514–527.

Butler, A. C., Karpicke, J. D., & Roediger, H. L. (2008). Correcting a metacognitive error: Feedback increases retention of low-confidence correct responses. *Journal of Experimental Psychology: Learning, Memory, and Cognition, 34*(4), 918–928.

Caputi, L., & Englemann, L. (2005*). Teaching nursing: The art and science.* Glen Ellyn, IL: College of DuPage Press.

Charania, N. A. M., Kauser, F., & Cassum, S. (2001). Educational innovations. Playing jigsaw: A cooperative learning experience. *Journal of Nursing Education, 40*(9), 420–421.

Cooper, C., & Carver, N. (2012). Problem based learning in mental health nursing: The students' experience. *International Journal of Mental Health Nursing, 21*(2), 175–183.

Cox-Davenport, R. A., & Phelan, J. C. (2015). Laying the groundwork for NCLEX success: An exploration of adaptive quizzing as an examination preparation method. *Computers, Informatics, Nursing, 33*(5), 208–215.

Duane, B. T., & Satre, M. E. (2014). Utilizing constructivism learning theory in collaborative testing as a creative strategy to promote essential nursing skills. *Nurse Education Today, 34* (1), 31–34.

Day, L. (2011). Using unfolding case studies in a subject-centered classroom. *Journal of Nursing Education, 50*(8), 447–452.

Eison, J. (2010). Using active learning instructional strategies to create excitement and enhance learning. Retrieved from http://www.cte.cornell.edu/documents/presentations/Eisen-Handout.pdf

Gagnon, L. L., & Roberge, G. D. (2011). Dissecting the journey: Nursing student experiences with collaboration during the group work process. *Nurse Education Today, 32*(8), 945–950.

Gallagher, P. A. (2009). Collaborative essay testing: Group work that counts. *International Journal of Nursing Education Scholarship, 6*(1), 1–13.

Hicks-Moore, S. L. (2005). Clinical concept maps in nursing education: An effective way to link theory and practice. *Nursing Education and Practice, 5* (6), 348–352.

Hubbard, G. B. (2014). Customized role play: Strategy for development of psychiatric mental health nurse practitioner competencies. *Perspectives in Psychiatric Care, 50*(2), 132–138.

Jigsaw.org (2015). History of the jigsaw. Retrieved from https://www.jigsaw.org/history/

Kinchin, I., & Hay, D. (2005). Using concept maps to optimize the composition of collaborative student groups: A pilot study. *Issues and Innovations in Nursing Education, 51* (2), 182–187.

Kung, D. T. (2013). Group work in college mathematics classes. Retrieved from http://collegemathvideocases.org/pdf/GroupWork.pdf

Krimshtein, N. S., Luhrs, C. A., Puntillo, K. A., Cortez, T. B., Livote, E. E., Penrol, J. D., & Nelson, J. E. (2011). Training nurses for interdisciplinary communication with families in the intensive care unit: An intervention. *Journal of Palliative Medicine, 14*(12), 1325–1332.

Novak, G. (2014). Just-in-time teaching: An interactive engagement pedagogy. Retrieved from http://www.edutopia.org/blog/just-in-time-teaching-gregor-novak

Novak, J. D., & Canas, A. J. (2008). The theory underlying concept maps and how to construct and use them. Retrieved from http://www.swwhs.org/site/wp-content/uploads/2013/06/2013-APPsychologySummerReadings.pdf

Orique, S. B., & McCarthy, M. A. (2015). Critical thinking and the use of nontraditional instructional methodologies. *Journal of Nursing Education, 54*(8), 455–459.

Purtee, M., Ulloth, J., & Caputi, L (2005). Developing and using case studies. In Caputi, L., & Engelmann, L (Eds.), *Teaching nursing: The art and science* (pp. 306–325). Glen Ellyn, IL: College of DuPage Press.

Samawi, Z. Miller, T., & Haras, M. S. (2014). Using high-fidelity simulation and concept mapping to cultivate self-confidence in nursing students. *Nursing Education Perspectives, 35*(6), 408–409.

Shin, H., Sok, S., Sun Hyun, K., & Kim, M. J. (2014). Competency and an active learning program in undergraduate nursing education. *Journal of Advanced Nursing, 71*(1), 591–598.

Shin, I., & Kim, J. (2013). The effect of problem-based learning in nursing education: A meta-analysis. *Advances in Health Science Education, 18*, 1103–1120.

Sim, S. M., Foong, C. C., Tan, C. H., Lai, P. S. M., Chua, S. S., & Mohazmi, M. (2014). The use of jigsaw learning technique in teaching medical students prescribing skills. *Medical Teacher, 36*(2), 182.

Thomas, T. G. (2009). *Active learning in encyclopedia of the social and cultural foundations of education*. Thousand Oaks, CA: SAGE Publications.

Trueman, G., Osuji, J., & El-Hussein, M. T. (2014). Baccalaureate nursing students' experience of dyadic learning in an acute care setting. *Journal of Nursing Education, 53*(9), S65–S72.

Ulrich, D., & Glendon, K. (1995). Jigsaw: A critical thinking experience. *Nurse Educator, 20*(3), 6–7.

Wong, C. K., & Driscoll, M. (2007). A modified jigsaw method: An active learning strategy to develop the cognitive and affective domains through curricular review. *Journal of Physical Therapy Education, 21*(3), 15–23.

CHAPTER 8

Did It Work? How to Evaluate Each Step of the Flipped Learning Environment

Introduction

The responsibilities of nursing educators expand beyond the planning and teaching of content into the realm of evaluation. Evaluation of teaching and learning in any profession can take on various forms and functions. Entire programs and curricula, courses, and individual student learning can all be the focus of evaluation efforts. This chapter will discuss evaluation of teaching and learning in the nursing education flipped classroom. Evaluation of instructor use of the pedagogy, evaluation of student preparation for in-class activities, and evaluation of student achievement of predetermined learning objectives will be discussed.

The idea of evaluation has been around for centuries. Evidence of the Chinese evaluating the functional capacity of civil servants has been discovered as early as 2000 B.C. (National Science Foundation, 2015). Some may think of evaluation only in the context of testing student knowledge or in terms of student evaluations of faculty at the end of a course. Although many definitions have been offered over the years, the Joint Committee on Standards for Educational Evaluation in 1994 defined evaluation as a "systematic investigation of the worth or merit of an object" (2015). Nurse educators Bourke and Ihrke (2005) have defined evaluation as "a means of appraising data or placing a value on data gathered through one or more measurements" (p. 443). For nursing education, these measurements focus on both the micro-level classroom and the macro-level program. Although flipped learning could be an adopted pedagogy for an entire curriculum, the focus of evaluation in this chapter will be on micro-level classroom and individual student learning evaluation.

Why is evaluation conducted? What is the purpose? Evaluation is valuable due to its ability to provide information or feedback that can help in a continuous improvement process. It can also offer new information not originally anticipated that changes the way business is conducted. In education, evaluation may also be applied to insuring student mastery of a subject. Mastery in one subject or class is often the key to the student's ability to move on to the next class or subject. Nursing curricula often use a stair step or pyramid approach to learning that requires students to have solid knowledge about one aspect of patient care before moving onto another. Subjects and courses often build upon one another in nursing programs. It would be illogical to allow a nursing student to take an advanced medical-surgical nursing class prior to showing proficiency in a pathophysiology or physical assessment course. On the contrary, the student must prove aptitude in pathophysiology and physical assessment courses before being allowed to continue the educational journey onto more complex topics including care of the critically ill patient. In this way, evaluation assists nurse educators in the important decision to allow a student's progression onto the next semester of content. It is an individual stamp of approval from one nurse educator to another to endorse student readiness for more complex and integrated content higher in the nursing curriculum pyramid.

Perhaps the first step of evaluation when considering the flipped classroom should focus on "business as usual" in the nursing education classroom. Why should flipped learning be considered as a vital pedagogy to nurse educators at all? As stated by Benner, Sutphen, Leonard, and Day (2010), there is a disconnect between what is taught in the classroom and what students experience in their clinical settings. Often considered the "theory-practice gap," the condition continues to persist in nursing education. What could be a solution to this condition that has been clearly identified by the intense research conducted in reflection of nursing education (Benner et al., 2010)? One solution presented by these authors included integrative teaching and learning. Included in this approach are ways to connect student clinical occurrences to the didactic learning picture. While it is impossible to be able to directly connect each student's clinical experience to what is being taught in the classroom, the authors offer expert advice for moving forward. There are simply too many diagnoses and individual patient scenarios to adequately capture each one in a timely manner in the didactic classroom environment. It would be impossible to know the future clinical experiences of each nursing student in order to write appropriate learning objectives and develop matching, applicable reading assignments. Nurse educators are largely stuck in the middle of the vast educational potential of the clinical setting, and the impossible task to teach students everything there is to know about it. The solution? Benner et al. have proposed use of integrative and interactive teaching and learning in the classroom that reflects the clinical atmosphere.

The flipped classroom can provide the interactive learning environment Benner and her colleagues have wisely suggested. When evaluating the current classroom pedagogy, consider how the worlds of clinical and theory are integrated. Are students being taught how to assimilate the learning in the classroom with what is learned in their clinical settings? Do clinical instructors know what is being taught in the classroom? Do classroom instructors know what is happening in the clinical settings? Is there congruency between what is learned in the clinical setting and what is learned in the classroom? Do students have a chance to individually think about and learn how to apply the content in the classroom to any given patient care scenario?

Does the classroom help prepare the student for their experiences in the clinical setting? Benner et al. (2010) recommend a classroom pedagogy that allows students to "imagine and rehearse how they might act in a clinical setting" (p. 160). Through case-based learning and problem-based solution discovery in the classroom, students can be assisted to develop a critical thinking paradigm from which to base patient care decisions. The flipped classroom allows not only time for this development to occur, but also a safe place with the additional benefit of immediate thought correction of the clinically expert nurse educator.

Evaluation of Student Learning in the Flipped Classroom

The rosters in nursing classrooms are fairly large. For this reason, many of the evaluation methods historically used by nurse educators have been "blanketed" approaches to assess student learning. Within this blanket approach is the typical exam or quiz, often with difficult advanced patient care knowledge questions used for the National Council Licensure Examination (NCLEX). It is not uncommon to hear nurse educators discuss the necessity of this type of testing in order to prepare students for the NCLEX exam that they will need to pass in order to legally practice their learned profession. This approach uses a micro-level assessment to prove proficiency of a more macro-level outcome. There exists a dichotomy of sorts when discussing this approach in nursing education. Nurse educators also commonly discuss the inappropriate educational approach of "teaching to the test" in the classroom. Although there is risk in expressing an inappropriate overarching generalization, it does appear that these are two very different opinions coming from the same professional group of educators. If nurse educators focus the majority of their evaluation efforts on exams in the classroom, how do they not teach to a test? These conflicting views leave some nurse educators with a lingering enigma about current and future approaches for the most valid and meaningful evaluation of student learning.

The Process of Evaluation

Bourke and Ihrke (2005) propose that evaluation is a process involving an organized sequence of actions. Identifying the purpose of the evaluation should be the first of these actions. *What is to be evaluated and why?* Clarity of this first step of the evaluation process is critical and can define many of the remaining actions of the process. Purposes for evaluation can be more narrow or broad in scope. Evaluation can be used to not only assess learning, but also facilitate learning. The idea of just-in-time teaching has at its core individual and group evaluation of understanding, or more specifically misunderstanding. Once the educator identifies the misconception of students, he or she is equipped to correct errors in thinking more readily. Students often don't know what they don't know. Therefore, educators must use evaluation of some sort to tease out this lack of knowledge and augment student learning in a meaningful way. Evaluation is often used as a way to measure knowledge level of student learning. Similarly, evaluation can be used to make a decision about student preparedness to continue on in a nursing program curriculum. In terms of the flipped classroom, evaluation can be used to assess student readiness for the in-class activities. It can also be helpful to assess faculty success with the method, or overall success in the classroom.

After clarifying what is to be evaluated and why, Bourke and Ihrke (2005) suggest identifying a time frame for the evaluation to occur. *Formative evaluation* (or assessment) is conducted during a program or learning activity. *Summative evaluation* refers to conducting evaluation at the end of the activity, pedagogy approach, course, or program. Some advantages to formative evaluation include an increase in the accuracy of the evaluation due to the immediacy of its occurrence. Less time goes by with formative assessment, allowing for a clearer and more "real-time" picture to evaluate. Results of the evaluation can also be used to guide or improve what is being evaluated on the spot. Just-in-time teaching uses such formative evaluation to guide the content discussed and taught in the flipped classroom environment.

Formative evaluation can also allow for important information about potential success or failure of what is being evaluated, which could be an enormous advantage. On the other hand, some disadvantages of formative assessment include conducting the evaluation with less information on hand. Conducting an evaluation with less information could lead to different outcomes than waiting to evaluate a product over time or at its summation. Formative evaluations also have the potential to disrupt the natural flow of the process being evaluated. A false sense of security with successful early evaluation could also be a disadvantage. For these reasons, formative assessment is typically used primarily as a feedback and continuous improvement process strategy in the classroom with students.

In a summative evaluation, the focus of evaluation includes a retrospective view of an entire event. The emphasis is on the extent to which any predetermined objectives and outcomes were met. In terms of timing, summative evaluation is conducted after an event occurs. Summative evaluation of student learning outcomes within a nursing course typically results in the assignment of a percentage and/or letter grade (Bourke & Ihrke, 2005). The main advantage of summative evaluation is the overarching retrospective view of any event being evaluated. All of the work and outcomes data are available for a complete global view from which evaluation can take place. Of course, the main disadvantage of summative evaluation is the lack of ability to alter or improve what is being evaluated. With summative evaluation, the event is indeed over and completed. Going back in time to change part of the event in order to improve the process or perhaps change the trajectory from failure to success is not possible.

The historical view of student learning evaluation in nursing has often come down to a summative opinion or quantitative evidence of either a pass or fail grade in individual courses and then the program in its entirety. Some educators may argue that giving several exams or quizzes throughout the semester offers a formative evaluation process. It could also be argued that once the exam has been given, it adds to the overall summative evaluation of student performance and cannot be changed. A more formative approach to evaluation can be achieved within the flipped classroom. Nurse educators are able to conduct mini-evaluations of student learning as they work with small groups and individual students more closely during the in-class sessions. Ability to conduct such formative assessment in the flipped classroom has the potential to change the summative evaluative approach to use of exams for measuring student learning outcomes.

Think for a moment about a student who has a solid understanding of the content when discussing it verbally. Is that same student's depth of knowledge revealed with use of a standardized exam? Could it be that the student really does have the knowledge necessary to carry out safe and effective patient care as a nurse, but has difficulty maneuvering an exam environment effectively? Additional challenges may occur for students from various cultures who may have a language barrier. Perhaps one can relate to the following scenario.

A student and nurse educator are meeting to discuss the student's poor performance on an exam. The faculty member realizes while talking with the student about the exam questions that the student really does have a good understanding of the content. Verbally, the student can easily meet the learning outcomes. The exam, for whatever reason, did not adequately reveal the student's knowledge base about the material. When faced with a multiple-choice format, the student was not able to choose the correct answer on a standardized test. There is a remaining question of how valid and reliable multiple-choice exam questions really are. Is this the most accurate measurement to evaluate student understanding of patient care concepts? It is uncertain if use of the flipped classroom will change the student's outcome on the same type of learning measurement. But it does have the potential to help the nurse faculty evaluate student learning in real time and correct errors in thinking. Deciding a more efficient and accurate way to measure knowledge level of student nurses will continue to be a question in need of additional attention and research.

Evaluation Practices With the Flipped Classroom

Evaluation of Off-Load Learning

Some nursing faculty who flip the classroom are interested in evaluating student knowledge of the off-load materials assigned. Many have voiced their belief of the necessity for students to prove their proficiency with the off-load material before they can be allowed to engage in the in-class learning activities. Some faculty have a differing opinion on the same topic. These faculty believe that the adult learner should rise to the occasion and become a responsible learner on his or her own. This approach typically means that students do not have to prove their proficiency with the off-load content. Instead, a culture is built in which completion of off-load assignments and activities to master lower-level objectives is a continual expectation. There is simply no other option in this culture of learning. The nursing student is viewed as an adult learner faced with an achievable task the student is expected to master. This culture teaches nursing students that learning does not happen without effort on their part.

The level of nursing students in the classroom may direct the nurse educator's approach to off-load assessment. Nursing educators who have flipped in both undergraduate and graduate courses have shared that the preparation for in-class activities can be dependent upon the level of student being taught. As one might expect, graduate-level nursing students are anecdotally much more likely to be prepared and able to self-regulate their off-load learning and preparation for in-class sessions. On the other hand, the undergraduate students may need more prompting or solid consequences for possible lack of preparation. These students are less likely to complete the off-load assignments, so it may be beneficial to plan for an assessment of off-load learning to insure that students are prepared for the in-class sessions.

Although building a culture of adult learning with a high expectation of preparation for in-class activities presents the educational utopia, it may be unrealistic. In-class activities are created using the higher-ordered learning objectives, and build upon the off-load objectives. Theoretically, if students have not completed the off-load assignments, they have not mastered those lower-ordered objectives and are not prepared to engage in higher-ordered learning. For this reason, many nurse educators would rather not leave the responsibility of preparation in the hands of the student. Requiring some sort of off-load assessment to show proficiency of the off-load learning objectives is often used by flipped-classroom nurse educators. Some of these strategies are quizzing, hand-in assignments, ticket-to-ride assignment, or short, student-led presentations.

Quizzing

The evaluation strategy of a short quiz to demonstrate student knowledge of off-load content is used by many flipped classroom instructors. The quiz can be in a paper-and-pencil or electronic format. Electronic-format quizzes are conducted with a classroom response system or using the learning management system. Several electronic student response systems are available. Most of the systems require each student to purchase a handheld response device that is compatible with the software used by the instructor. Many colleges and universities have adopted a specific type of classroom response system to be used campus wide. When this approach is used, students at that university only have to buy one response device during their time at that particular institution. Some schools or colleges of nursing have purchased a set of student response devices for their program. When educators want to use the classroom response system, they hand out the devices to individual students who have been assigned a device number. The devices are relatively inexpensive in the world of costly technology, with a price hovering around $40 to $50 each. The fact that students can use the same clicker over and over in different classes makes this purchase a bit more reasonable. Some response systems use the students' cellular phones and text messaging. Although this initially seems like a great idea, the tactic leaves the student without a cell phone out of the quizzing picture.

The response device is considered a book purchase if required by the course, and therefore can be covered by most if not all financial aid and scholarship dollars.

Another great innovation to use in place of a more costly student response system can be found free online. Nolan Amy, a math teacher in Richmond, California, and colleagues created a response system using paper cards for students that can be scanned by the instructor using any mobile device (Plickers.com, 2015). Faculty simply sign in for a free account, download and print out a set of plickers and then download the plickers app on their mobile device. After logging in on a personal computer, questions can be added to a class that is created by the instructor. Once in the classroom, each student is given a plicker (printed out individually from the website). The instructor selects which question they want the students to answer on the app, and then use their camera feature to scan the audience of students. Students simply move their plicker card to show their chosen answer at the top of the scanned plicker. It might seem like something so low tech would not be effective, but the plickers work amazingly well. Better yet, students love the plickers because they are fun and free!

When used as an evaluation method for off-load learning, quizzes are typically short. Most faculty report that these quizzes contain between 7 to 10 questions focused on the off-load learning objectives. Quizzing does offer the nursing instructor with some assurance of individual student's engagement with the off-load assignments. Particularly when the quizzes are used as a part of the students' overall grade, students are more likely to be motivated to learn the content prior to coming to class. Some flipping educators have even had students complete a graded quiz on the learning management system online prior to coming to class for up to 60% of the total grade (Critz & Knight, 2013). There may be a few flaws in this evaluation approach. Can a short quiz of 10 questions or less really capture student understanding of off-load content to the level of mastery? Perhaps the quiz can show some level of student proficiency, which provides a valuable nugget of assurance for nursing faculty. Difficulty creating standardized questions that reflect a true measurement of student knowledge level continues to be a challenge.

Some nursing faculty use the quizzes as only a teaching and learning tool. In this scenario, no points are allocated for quizzing outcomes. Students can learn more about the material question by question, allowing for formative assessment and self-reflection of knowledge. Educators have been able to work with the just-in-time teaching approach together with the quizzing strategy to correct errors in thinking with immediate feedback from faculty (McLaughlin et al., 2014). The downside to this approach is the lack of true individual assessment of student knowledge of the off-load material assigned. Students could get answers wrong on the quizzes due to lack of preparation and have no real consequences. It does seem that when quizzing is used as a teaching strategy rather than an evaluation method, student learning is augmented for both the prepared and unprepared student.

Hand-In Assignments

Some flipping faculty use a number of assignments that students must hand in to show proficiency with off-load material. Depending on the class and the content to be mastered, the faculty may have students work individually or in groups on such assignments. The assignment must be completed prior to coming to class, and handed in prior to the in-class session beginning. One example is a simple worksheet for students to complete to show their understanding of the off-load objectives. An example of a very simple handout for teaching lower-level objectives about common male testicular conditions is provided in **Figure 8-1**. In this example, students are asked to complete part of the worksheet for the off-load assignment. Each student is to bring the partially completed worksheet to class where the remainder is completed in small groups. After the worksheet has been completed by all groups, a short teaching session is conducted in which groups share their information and questions are answered. The next step for the in-class session is a complex case study. Students use the information that they've completed on the

Name	(1) Etiology	(2) Common Symptoms	(3) Physical Exam	(4) Differential Dx	(5) Treatment
Epididymitis					
Testicular Torsion					
Testicular CA					
Viral Orchitis					

Instructions: After completing the assigned readings and watching the assigned video content for the unit, complete individually columns (1) Etiology and (2) Common Symptoms. Bring your assignment to class where we will be working to complete the remaining columns in class.

Figure 8-1 Example of a hand-in assignment.

worksheet and apply it to a case-based or problem-based scenario in their small groups.

Other strategies for hand-in assignments include completion of a charting exercise, synopsis of a research article, or a vocabulary worksheet. It may seem childlike for some, but completion of crossword puzzles can be used as a strategy to show competency in rote memorization of terms. There are some great websites available for creation of crossword puzzles. One that is often used by nurse educators can be found on The Teacher's Corner at the following URL: http://www.theteacherscorner.net. This particular site also has some other free worksheet templates for educators, such as write-in worksheets and other vocabulary games. When brought to class, each of these will prove some level of proficiency with the off-load material. Whether or not to give points for these type of activities that count toward the final grade is decided by instructor preference.

Ticket to Ride

The ticket to ride is a short assignment created by educators to demonstrate individual student knowledge of the off-load learning objectives. Such an approach can encourage the students to complete off-load assignments as assigned and therefore prepare them for the in-class activities. It is termed a *ticket to ride* because students need to hand it in prior to being let into the in-class session, much like the ticket necessary prior to paid transportation. A hand-in worksheet as mentioned previously may serve the purpose of the ticket to ride. Ticket to ride can be complex or simple. For example, when discussing chronic illness, have the students bring in a picture that speaks chronic illness to them. Just bringing a picture shows that they've invested some time in thinking about their view of chronic illness. It is also a strategy of some nurse educators to embed the ticket-to-ride assignment into their video. Within the video lecture, the nurse educator will tell students what they will need to bring to class for ticket to ride. If they bring the ticket-to-ride item mentioned in the video, it is apparent that the video was at the very least viewed by the student.

A lingering question connected to ticket to ride is what to do if the student does not bring the ticket to ride. What will be the consequence, if any? Once again, this is largely left up to educator preference. Some educators give students one "oops" or "pass" a semester to not bring the ticket to ride. Others allocate points to the ticket to ride in order to strongly encourage students complete the assignment and bring their ticket to ride. Again, educators teaching in an undergraduate program may find more value in attaching a consequence such as loss of points in the course for failing to bring the ticket to ride. To summarize, *ticket to ride* denotes a term that encompasses any number of off-load assignments that students must turn in at the beginning of an in-class session.

Allow me to share some lessons learned using the ticket-to-ride concept. In the real world of flipped learning, the off-load assessments of learning can produce more work for both students and educators that I am not certain are terribly advantageous. If the biggest pedagogical advantage of the flipped classroom is spending the live, face-to-face time with students in a more engaging manner, do we really want to use the first 15 or 20 minutes of that live class time grading off-load assessment of learning assignments? Realistically, when we used the ticket to ride, we mostly took a quick glance to be certain the sheet of paper had been completed by each individual student. Later when we had the time, we went back and did a more thorough job of grading those assignments. When used in this manner, the off-load assessment of learning is really only used as an insurance policy that students have done something with the off-load materials, not a measurement of their learning prior to in-class activities.

Student-Led Presentations

It is not uncommon for faculty to use preparation of student-led presentations as an off-load assignment. Whether individually or in a group, students must be prepared during the in-class session to present part or all of the prepared product about a certain topic. The student presentation offers a chance for evaluation of student understanding and completion of off-load assignments. Along that same line of assumptions, students who have prepared content to present to the class or perhaps within their small group are likely to be prepared for additional in-class learning. The act of presenting the material during the in-class session is controversial. Peer instruction can be valuable if done correctly by peers who have taken time and attention to develop a discussion or argument for their classmates. The main concern with this method may be that it takes interactive learning out of the equation. Other than the student who is presenting, there is little to no interactivity in student-led presentations. Although it does provide that evaluation piece that can be valuable to nurse educators, it puts lecture back on the main stage of learning. The only difference is that the student is delivering the lecture rather than the instructor, which has its own host of challenges.

Evaluation of Instructor Use of the Flipped Classroom

Being a new pedagogy for most nurse educators, evaluating use of the method can be extremely helpful for revision and refinement. Included within this evaluation are how the educator prepared students for the pedagogy, how they were able to create the off-load assignments to match the in-class activities, and their management of in-class activity time. Evaluation of individual instructor use of the pedagogy can be achieved with a few strategies. It is difficult if not impossible to evaluate oneself in an objective manner. For this reason, asking for assistance with the evaluation of instructor effectiveness is beneficial. Finding faculty who have flipped successfully to help evaluate the process can be extremely beneficial. At this time there are no research-validated evaluation tools for use of the flipped classroom. One might consider using the Intentional Instruction Model to assist in evaluating each piece of a faculty member's flipped classroom in a structured manner.

Finding another nursing faculty member to evaluate your flipped classroom may be a challenge at this point in time because there are not many out there flipping. There are, however, more and more faculty across disciplines flipping their classroom on any given university campus. It is completely acceptable to go outside the discipline of nursing to find other flipping faculty to help evaluate the flipping process itself. Use of faculty colleagues in math has proven to be very helpful for a clear view of my own flipping practices. The same colleagues are teaching me how to refine my techniques and tactics when flipping the classroom. The flipped classroom model is transferrable between very different disciplines in that it is not content specific. Several years back I had a colleague from the statistics department evaluate my teaching in the classroom for purposes of the tenure process. We were also helping to develop a peer faculty evaluation of teaching tool for our campus. The experience provided me with so many excellent ideas. It also gave me a very clear and unbiased view of myself as an instructor—as a nurse or a nurse practitioner, but as an educator. I would encourage this type of cross-discipline evaluation for everyone. Asking a seasoned faculty member from outside your own discipline can be a very valuable evaluative strategy.

Similar to having a colleague critique your use of the method, take the time to visit the classroom of a flipping colleague. Once again, the class content does not need to focus on nursing. The focus of the visit would be to watch how other faculty use the flipped classroom, engage students in the learning activities during class, and manage their class time effectively. It may also be helpful to schedule a short meeting with your peer after the visitation to their classroom. Ask any questions that came up as you watched the class unfold. Ask your peer how he or she assesses the class management and for a rationale of his or her teaching strategy. Objective peer evaluation can be very informative, but much can be learned from peer observation as well.

Although it may be a bit less objective, self-evaluation can be conducted on the use of the flipped classroom. It can provide valuable avenues for revision and refinement. By and large, educators tend to be too hard on themselves and need that peer view to balance their more critical view of their own performance. Use of a self-reflection journal completed right after the process can help to capture some raw data on success or difficulty using the method. Nurse educators are often too busy to take the time to stop and reflect on their class time and teaching strategies. Particularly right after the flipped classroom is used, sit down to think about what went well and what could have run more smoothly. Brainstorm about ways to better the process for the next time the flipped classroom will be implemented. Review the learning objectives for the off-load and in-class activities to see if any were missed. Were students prepared for the in-class activities at a high enough competency level? Did the off-load assignments assist in this preparation? Perhaps there were some off-load assignments that never made it into the in-class learning session that could be deleted.

For example, when first flipping, a colleague was using the video lecture and typical readings from the student textbook. She also loaded four to five research-based articles about the content that she thought would be of interest and add to student learning of the content and preparation for the in-class session. Upon reflection, she realized that although she wanted the students to have an appreciation for evidence-based practice, she was not using any of the research articles in the in-class session. The articles may have been a good idea initially, but it was found that they did not really add anything in terms of increasing student understanding. They did, however, overwhelm the students with more off-load content to review. As one might imagine, student resistance to the amount of off-load materials assigned was also a problem. The solution? She took the articles out of the off-load materials in favor of using them as supporting evidence for class discussions. She also used the articles for student groups to read and discuss in the event that the in-class activities ran short.

While engaging in self-reflection, take a close look at the learning objectives for your flipped classroom. Sometimes nurse educators are surprised when they do so. There is not typically a problem with educators not covering the written objectives for the unit or course. More often, it is the opposite scenario of going above and beyond teaching the students what is written in the learning objectives. At times, educators feel like they can't get through or teach all of the content expected in a particular course. A closer look may reveal that faculty who feel very passionate about a subject will augment and expand the original objectives without even realizing they are doing so. One faculty member may see a unit entitled "high-risk obstetrics" and use the learning objectives as a definitive guide for instructional content. Another faculty member who has a passion for obstetrical nursing may see the same unit and begin to conjure up in his or her mind all the student needs to know about that particular content according to his or her own educational compass. I feel comfortable writing about this because I am guilty of this very thing. I have additional education, training, and clinical experience as an obstetrical nurse and nurse practitioner. It is personally difficult for me to reign in my passion and knowledge about this content when teaching the undergraduate nursing student who needs to know a fraction of what I think the student needs to know. Some nurse educators may not relate to this scenario at all, but I am guessing that there may be a few that can resonate with this notion. It is a very helpful evaluation tool to do a self-check of what actually occurs in the classroom teaching and learning environment with what the learning objectives say should be occurring. Although this step of evaluation is not unique to the flipped classroom, it is certainly an important one.

Once a self-reflection or peer evaluation of the flipped classroom has taken place, revisions need to occur. This may go without saying for many readers, but it is highly recommended that the flipping nurse educator implement changes right away. Even if the class will not be taught again until the next year, make any suggested changes as soon as possible. Too often the excellent feedback on how to revise is forgotten and only remembered when teaching the class again. Take the time to work on those changes before they escape the mind and become a distant memory.

Summative evaluations of educators by their students have historically been used as a main tool for evaluation of teaching assessment in the nursing education classroom. In an integrative review of the literature, Annan, Tratnack, Rubenstein, Metzler-Sawin, and

Hulton (2013) attempted to summarize the current literature about the use of student evaluations of nursing instructors. There is a question of the validity and reliability of many student evaluation tools being used in programs to grasp a clear picture of true faculty abilities in teaching and learning. The authors discussed the various roles in which faculty teach students including classroom, simulation labs, and clinical settings. Seeing faculty in a variety of education roles may confuse student responses on evaluation tools. Perhaps the largest concern is that most, if not all, of the evaluation tools used are homemade, lacking true validity and reliability data.

Overall, the integrative review supported that educators are divided in their views about the usability, reliability, and validity of student evaluations (Annan et al., 2013). Some faculty interpret student evaluations of faculty as a measure of popularity rather than excellence in teaching. Educators do seem to agree that students are not pedagogical experts and their evaluation of educator effectiveness should be viewed with this lens. Of interest, students rated educator higher on evaluations when they perceived the educator as being experienced, clear, enthusiastic, helpful, fair, and organized. Although these are helpful characteristics to manage a classroom effectively, they are not directly related to the educator's teaching ability. Perhaps a more accurate measurement of educator success could be student learning outcomes. Of course, use of student outcome data can be flawed in terms of validity and reliability itself. Getting to the heart of the matter and truly answering the question of educators' teaching ability is much more complex than it seems. Couple these issues with the fact that student evaluations are used by many universities as a measuring stick for faculty promotion, tenure, and merit. It is clear that higher education has a great deal of work to do in the realm of evaluation in general. Nursing education is no different.

The point of this discussion is that student evaluations of educators' teaching need to be considered in light of their true ability to reflect excellence in teaching. The reality is that students are students. They often cannot appreciate the complexity involved in the teaching and learning experience to the point of being capable of providing valid assessments of teaching effectiveness. Shift thought for a moment to the world of nursing. A patient has had a total hip replacement and is now in your nursing care. Even though the patient's pain has been managed effectively, he is resistant to ambulation. What is the role of the nurse? Is it to do what the patient desires in order to gain favor with the patient? Most (if not all) would agree that the role of the nurse is to ambulate the patient. Doing so reflects the nurse's knowledge that ambulation stimulates circulation, prevents pneumonia, slowly increases mobility, and promotes ultimate recovery. The patient may not be particularly happy about having to ambulate, but ambulation is what the patient needs. After patient recovers, the patient is thankful to the nurse for putting the patient's needs above his or her more immediate comfort and desires. The nurse holds knowledge about patient care that the patient cannot fully appreciate. When shifting thought back to the classroom, can a mirror image be seen? Do the teaching strategies used align more with what the students want or what the students need? Could it be that educators are gravitating toward student satisfaction more than they are effective teaching? It is difficult for educators to be diligent in their goal to educate rather than placate. The pressure to placate is very real, particularly when student evaluations are used as a main measure of teaching ability with the potential to effect tenure and promotion.

There is one last thought about instructor evaluation of the flipped classroom. *Don't be too hard on yourself.* It is normal for students to show resistance (a little and sometimes a lot) to use of the flipped classroom. Try to recall the research reviewed earlier in the text matching several anecdotal accounts that students do get used to flipping over time. Most do not like the method to begin with and that is okay. It is more work and requires that students move outside of their comfort zone in the classroom. Try to resist the urge to switch back to straight lecture. Students really do appreciate the ability to make their learning more interactive, but it takes them a while to recognize that appreciation and express it. Some students will hold out and not be accepting of the method at all. It takes them a while to realize that they are not only learning the content, but moving their understanding of the content into a deeper realm of practical understanding. Our classrooms should reflect the idea that nursing is not a spectator sport.

Conclusion

The topic of evaluation often brings more questions than answers to light. It is clear that finding valid and reliable evaluation tools to measure effectiveness of the flipped classroom on many levels may be a challenge. Use of standardized exams will most likely continue to be the mainstream evaluation method for measurement of student knowledge outcomes in nursing programs. Although testing has its flaws, it seems to be a widely used tool in the world of nursing evaluation. It is no secret that additional research is needed to make informed decisions about the most effective way to move forward to evaluate student learning with the use of the flipped classroom. Use of the flipped classroom may prove to be more effective in knowledge retention in nursing students. At this point, there is no research to support or refute this idea.

Much of the existing research has used student test or exam scores in a before-and-after use of the classroom research design. Often, the results show better grades in the flipped classroom but not at a statistically significant level. Perhaps finding statistically significant differences in exams and final grades with nursing students will not be an attainable research goal. By and large, nursing students are a highly motivated and intelligent group. Small increases in knowledge may not be statistically measurable when all grades are higher to begin with. Finding a worthy and meaningful way to measure the effectiveness of the flipped classroom will continue to be a challenge for education researchers.

Until the state of the science expands to inform practices in the classroom, it is worth time and effort to evaluate use of the method in more practical ways. Use of educator peer review of the method can be helpful in many ways. Asking students their views can be informative, but also a slippery slope to maneuver. It is not uncommon for faculty to become discouraged when asking students for their opinion too early in their experience of the flipped classroom. Until more formal research is available for guidance, the nurse educator must rely on the feedback of those intimately involved in the process. These feedback resources include the students, other flipping faculty, and a healthy dose of self-reflection.

References

Annan, S. L., Tratnack, S., Rubenstein, C. Metzler-Sawin, E., & Hulton, L. (2013). An integrative review of student evaluations of teaching: Implications for evaluation of nursing faculty. *Journal of Professional Nursing, 29*(5), e10–e24.

Benner, P., Sutphen, M., Leonard, V., & Day, L. (2010). *Education nurses: A call for radical transformation.* Stanford, CA: The Carnegie Foundation for the Advancement of Teaching.

Bourke, M. P., & Ihrke, B. A. (2005). The evaluation process and overview. In D. M. Billings & J. A. Halstead (Eds.), *Teaching in nursing: A guide for faculty* (2nd ed., pp. 443–464). St. Louis, MO: Elsevier.

Critz, C. M., & Knight, D. (2013). Using the flipped classroom in graduate nursing education. *Nurse Educator, 38*(5), 210–213.

McLaughlin, J. E., Roth, M. T., Glatt, D. M., Gharkholonarehe, N., Davidson, C. A., Griffin, L. M., Esserman, D. A., & Mumper, R. J. (2014). The flipped classroom: A course redesign to foster learning and engagement in a health professions school. *Academic Medicine, 89*(2), 1–8.

National Science Foundation. (2015). Evaluation and types of evaluation. Retrieved from http://www.nsf.gov/pubs/2002/nsf02057/nsf02057_2.pdf

Plickers.com. (2015). About Plickers. Retrieved from https://plickers.com/about

CHAPTER 9

Those Flipping Nursing Instructors!

Introduction

There are a few nurse educators who have implemented the flipped classroom across our nation and around the world. I am so very fortunate that a few of these excellent educators have been willing to share their ideas and experiences with the flipped classroom to include within this chapter. I think you will find some excellent and creative ideas from each of their experiences. It is my hope that each of the following flipped classroom exemplars will inspire you to create your own brand and flavor of flipped learning that you will also share with your fellow nurse educators someday.

Katherine (Kat) Johnson, MSN, CPNP

Kat Johnson is a Pediatric Nurse Practitioner and previous Assistant Professor of Nursing at the University of Northern Colorado (UNC) School of Nursing. Although she recently left nursing education to pursue her love of pediatric clinical practice, she taught graduate and undergraduate pediatrics for a little over 8 years. Kat and I were the first nurse educators to flip the classroom on our campus. We learned many lessons in that first experience, which Kat was able to develop more fully into her undergraduate pediatrics nursing courses. Her ideas for the active learning phase of the flipped classroom are extremely innovative and fun, but also carefully designed to keep everyone's focus on learning. Kat embodies the perfect combination of skillful practitioner and natural scholar, so I am most grateful she has chosen to share a little bit about her process of flipping the classroom for all of us to learn from.

When Kat began flipping her pediatrics nursing course, she found that the students had never been exposed to the pedagogy in their previous courses. For this reason, she was careful to educate students about the pedagogy, including student expectations, and how the flipped classroom is different from the previous experience of straight lecture. Like many other flipping nursing instructors have reported, Kat explained that some of her students were positive about the process, while others were consistently negative. Having been the chair of the undergraduate curriculum committee, Kat was very knowledgeable about concept-based curriculum. The school of nursing at UNC did not use a concept-based curriculum at the time of this printing. However, Kat did teach concepts first in her pediatric class, followed by disease states, which were then connected to associated medical and nursing care.

Kat mentioned that with her experience using the flipped classroom and the extensive research she had engaged in for her role as curriculum chair, the flipped classroom presented an excellent pedagogy to use within a concept-based curriculum. One of the reasons for the flipped classroom's natural fit with concept-based teaching is the ability to review content from previous weeks during in-class sessions. With concept-based teaching, the tie-in of each concept from week to week would provide a natural review and reapplication of the material. In Kat's mind, this would be an excellent way to not only teach the material, but also allow the students to scaffold new learning onto existing long-term memory. The way that students can make connections from what was learned to what needs to be learned introduces the cognitive load theory principle of a schema. For a review of cognitive load theory, see **Box 9-1**.

When first flipping the classroom, Kat recorded many of her own lectures for off-load, but also used videos she found on the Internet.

BOX 9-1 Cognitive Load Theory Review

- Working memory load can be described as the mental effort necessary to accomplish a task or tasks, and may be affected by both the *intrinsic cognitive load* and *extraneous cognitive load* (Sweller, van Merrienboer, & Paas, 1998).
  - **Intrinsic cognitive load** is concerned with the level of difficulty of the information that must be understood and learned and cannot be altered (Sweller, 2010).
    - The way in which students are taught affects the way they process information in working memory and store information in long-term memory for recall at a later point.
  - **Extraneous cognitive load** is the load imposed on the learner by instructional design or how the material is presented to the learner (Swellar).
- Intrinsic cognitive load is determined by the complexity of material presented, while the extraneous cognitive load, the way in which the material is presented to the students, can be altered.
  - The intrinsic load of nursing education material is typically high and therefore requires an effort on the part of the nursing instructor to help the student learn by lowering of extraneous cognitive through improved instructional design efforts such as active/interactive learning in the flipped classroom.
- **Schema construction** promotes student storage of data points in long-term memory and assists in the learning and retention of material.
- Students "scaffold" new information onto existing long-term memory, which aids in retention of the material in the long-term memory or true learning of the material.
  - *Example: The student understands the way a plumbing system works; using this previous knowledge, the signs and symptoms of congestive heart failure can be taught using the pre-existing knowledge about how plumbing works.*

After more experience with flipping and constructive student feedback, she found that she posted fewer of her own lectures and recordings for off-load assignments. Kat agreed with the previously mentioned "off-load mastery learning" concept, discussing that a few of her students were able to judge just how much they needed to view/complete prior to coming to class rather than feeling that they had to view all content regardless of their own knowledge base. We discussed that it does take students time to trust the flipping instructor in the assigning of off-load content. Nursing students (and maybe students in general) tend to be nervous that they will miss something assigned, and compensate by over-doing things at times. Herein lies the danger of assigning too many off-load materials and expecting students to self-regulate their own learning. Mastery learning for off-load content is certainly something that needs further exploration and consideration within the flipped classroom model. We need some solid research and/or advice on how to teach our students this mastery process or learning self-regulation. It does come naturally for some, while others tend to struggle with their ability to gauge their individual needs in terms of learning the objectives for the course.

The discussion of using pre-made videos from a variety of sources for assignment in the off-load reminded Kat of a careful suggestion for fellow flipping educators. Although using others' videos and work is beneficial, caution is recommended. Finding videos that fit the learning objectives at hand can be very time consuming. After an exhaustive search on the Internet, there may not be a video that captures what you want to teach your students. It is therefore important to remember that finding these types of off-load sources takes time and patience. If you don't find exactly what you are looking for in a pre-made video within the first 15 minutes of a search, it is likely not out there. Instead of a frustrating search or posting a video that is not exactly what you wanted, try to remember your course content as you see things here and there on various sources of media that might be perfect for implementation within your flipped classroom.

Allow me to provide an example of what is described above. In my own flipped classroom, I teach a unit on geriatric health promotion. Students have in their off-load assignment several excellent short lecture videos created by a brilliant graduate student who is also a geriatric nurse practitioner. After she recorded the videos, we saw a great *60 Minutes* episode on aging and staying healthy, including some extremely well-done and meaningful research that added to our original materials. We kept the lecture videos, but added these new ones to the off-load assignments.

I was expecting the students to be upset with the additional content to view during the off-load but forgot two critical things that were in my favor. The first is that these students had no prior reference of what was assigned for that unit, and therefore did not know that there were "additional" videos. The second was that the content was so well done and meaningful that students reported absolutely enjoying the *60 Minutes* videos assigned. The videos also brought about a nice connection to the previously recorded lecture videos, all of which brought about an excellent in-class discussion and application session.

When Kat found Internet videos for her students, they were not focused on what you might typically expect. The assigned videos always added to the readings and lecture slides or videos in some way and did not repeat any content. Instead, she provided the example of using videos posted on the Internet of children with the disease states and/or of their parents telling their stories. Students used their readings, the short video lecture or review of previous lecture slides, and the video to form a 3-dimensional picture if you will, of the disease state. Instead of only thinking about signs and symptoms, Kat wanted students to watch the signs and symptoms and be able to pick them out of the videos she assigned. She wanted her students to gain an affective understanding of what the child and parents have gone through on their disease journey. Then she connected all of this information back to the expected medical care and nursing interventions for a patient and family with a similar condition within the face to face or in-class time with the pediatric students.

As Kat gained more experience with the flipped classroom, she began to post her lecture slides without notes or video for students to simply use as a study guide. The videos that she assigned along with these lecture slides were used to augment rather than repeat any material as mentioned above. She also attempted to match her off-load and in-class assignments and activities to the different learning styles of all students. Some are more visual, while others learn more effectively through auditory or verbal cues, and still others are more tactile learners. In Kat's flipped classroom, there was a teaching and learning approach for everyone in the room. I admire this in Kat's teaching style. It takes a great deal of time and planning to be certain all learning styles are accommodated. I will admit that I have not spent as much time thinking about this aspect of teaching and learning that I no doubt should. Kat reminds me that flipping the classroom allows for this type of tailor-made classroom. With practice and commitment, each student's own learning style can be provided to enhance their individual understanding of the material at hand. Perhaps Kat is showing us yet another way to think about mastery of learning; mastery for each student via attention to each individual's learning style.

As mentioned earlier, Kat's interactive in-class time was legendary. She had a way of creating activities for students in both groups and as individuals that drive home the learning of any material in a unique and creative way. She had one of those personalities that makes everything fun, and students loved her classes, flipped or not. Kat used quite a few case studies for her in-class application sessions. After putting the students into groups of 4 to 8 depending on the topic, she would assign each group to prepare a short teaching session for their fellow students on one aspect of the topic. As recommended in the flipped classroom, these topics were focused on the application of off-load materials, and generally focused around the associated medical orders and nursing interventions.

Using the "jig-saw," Kat had the groups re-organize so that the new groups had one person from each teaching topic in one group. As the students moved around the room, the student who helped create the teaching material taught the others in the newly formed group. The jig-saw is a bit confusing to grasp initially, but was an extremely effective interactive learning strategy once in motion. Each student must teach the content one time, and making students teach content, as we know, is a highly efficacious learning strategy. In another class on communicable diseases, Kat had the students form a teaching plan for parents regarding the risks of the illness, signs and symptoms, and vaccines with associated side effects. Students could use their resources and computers to access information to complete these teaching materials. She had the students teach their content to the other students, sometimes using the jig-saw and other times having each group go to the front of the class to teach their information to the rest of the students. Putting students in the role of teacher not only augments their own learning, but also gets them prepared to step into the role of patient and family educator.

Kat mentioned that when she used case studies in her flipped classroom she always did so in a different and fresh way for each in-class period. At times she would provide students the admission diagnosis, previous nurse's report, and patient assessment information in the first part of the case study. The students were then assigned a set of labs to interpret and develop appropriate nursing actions. Other times she provided the students with only the patient demographics, and signs and symptoms or history of present illness. She then assigned the students to think of different disease processes that might fit that picture. Still another approach was to offer the students only the disease state and have them think of signs and symptoms and most common demographics associated. For all of these different approaches, the final step of the process always culminated in students fleshing out the expected medical orders, appropriate nursing interventions, and salient patient and family teaching associated with the disease state.

One particular case study Kat shared was focused on a type 1 diabetic adolescent athlete with diabetic ketoacidosis (DKA). Students learned the concepts of type 1 diabetes with DKA in their off-load assignments. Once they came to class, Kat assigned the case study to student groups focusing on sick day management for the patient described in the case study. After the students completed the case study, the answers were reviewed as a group. During the discussion period, Kat used just-in-time teaching techniques that matched the students' understanding. The next part of the in-class time was spent with student groups considering how the sick day management would be different for a toddler or school-aged child. The ability for students to transfer what was learned about sick day management with the adolescent provided an important learning activity. Allowing students to gain some solid understanding of nursing interventions for one age group and then requiring them to transfer that knowledge to another age group allowed for schema development. Schema development, in turn, allows for enhanced learning ability.

Still another of Kat's flipped classes helped students to gain a deeper understanding of pediatric growth and development with a very inventive instructional design. The off-load included readings and the assignment for each student to bring to class a picture of an age and developmentally appropriate toy for a pre-assigned age group. Students had to discuss with the class why they chose the toy, how it was appropriate for specified age group, and how it assisted the child in reaching a specific developmental milestone. As you can imagine, the direct application of toys to age and developmental milestone provided a more rounded picture of growth and development. Instead of thinking about growth and development within the typical linear fashion, Kat was able to move students into the world of pediatric growth and development with a direct application of material. The ability for the students to provide their pediatric patients the correct toys in their clinical, and the aptitude to teach parents about developmentally appropriate toys were additional benefits of this exercise.

Kat has also used concept maps in both her off-load and in-class assignments. Many times, the concept maps are done in a group and used for the jig-saw teaching strategy mentioned earlier. Another visual exercise Kat used involved students drawing a disease state without any words. She typically used this exercise when she taught endocrine disorders. In the off-load, students had the lower-ordered objectives of reviewing the pathophysiology and signs and symptoms. In class, each student was given a small sheet of paper with a disease state written on it. The student would then use a blank sheet of paper to draw the disease. Then without using anything but the picture, students would show their picture to either their group of the entire class (depending on the size of the class). The class would use only the picture to guess what the disease state was. The next part of class used these pictures to develop nursing diagnoses and interventions associated with each disease state.

Yet another in-class activity Kat used often was a bit like gaming. At the beginning of the class as they entered, each student was given a small slip of paper with a symptom written on it. Using the example of respiratory conditions, the symptoms would be "shortness of breath," "low oxygen saturation," "dizziness," "wheezing," and so on. The students were then asked to congregate to disease states that were posted on the walls of the classroom. Kat called this teaching strategy "symptom, symptom, who's got a symptom." She mentioned that this could be initially thought of as a lower-ordered learning activity, but quickly reminded that the ability for students to think abstractly about the symptoms and where they should be located included the higher-ordered skill of analysis. This activity was followed by a class discussion of what nursing interventions would be attached to each symptom, how they were similar and different from one another, and how the nurse would react differently with the symptom occurring in different age groups of pediatric patients.

Although Kat had become an expert at the flipped classroom, there were still times that she chose lecture as the most appropriate teaching strategy. She chose to lecture about pediatric cardiac conditions due to general student confusion about this topic, and inability of students to grasp a deep enough understanding about the conditions themselves during the off-load assignments. Although students have learned about these conditions in their pathophysiology courses, the amount of time spent on the content is generally very scant. For this reason, Kat found that a solid lecture period to be in front of the classroom to visually engage the students with her hands-on explanation of each cardiac condition was necessary. Knowing the way Kat teaches, there was an expectation of student interaction, questions, and responses from the group of students in the classroom seats.

Like many nurse educators, Kat taught courses in the graduate and undergraduate programs simultaneously. She mentioned that she was careful to consider the level of learner in her classroom while planning the flipped classroom. Strategies that work well for undergraduate nursing students do not automatically transfer to success with graduate students. Admittedly, an understanding of which things were best for each group took some time, trial, and error. Kat recommended a continual focus on learning objectives to help design the flipped classroom. The learning objectives should provide that road map for planning and ultimate success. For example, if undergraduate pediatric nursing students are to learn bedside hospital nursing interventions for low blood sugar, the graduate nursing student objective may be more focused on recognizing how to diagnose blood sugar abnormalities in the primary care setting. Paying close attention to those learning objectives and the diverse audience of students in each classroom will allow for a more appropriate instruction design of any flipped classroom.

We can all learn so much from Kat's flipped classroom exemplar (see **Box 9-2** for her flip tips). I would like to thank her for embarking on the original flipped classroom journey with me. It has been so much fun working with her and sharing ideas, presenting on the flipped classroom, and supporting one another during the process. Kat is one of those women that just shines in any role. Thank you, Kat, for helping us understand the brilliance and dedication within your flipped classroom, and sharing a bit of your ingenuity for us to emulate!

BOX 9-2 Kat's Flip Tips

- If you don't at first succeed, don't give up! The flipped classroom really works, but does take some practice and refining.
- If students don't come prepared, let them have a "do-over." Have a discussion with them about the necessity of being prepared and email to put it in writing.
- Give some points for off-load assignments and in-class engagement, but only around 10%.
- Adapt to the specific learning needs of your flipped classroom students – second-degree students might need different activities and assignments than traditional nursing students.
- Assign students to groups for in-class group work, switch up the groups during the semester, and expose students to different personalities to simulate the true nursing environment they will soon experience.
- Keep the size of student groups smaller to increase productivity and engagement of each student.
- Listen to student feedback and use it to fine tune your flipped classroom – but be able to discern constructive criticism from good, old-fashioned complaining.
- Find a way to weave content the students have learned earlier in the semester back into the current learning activities. Help students make connections and use abstract and critical thinking skills to deepen their understanding.

Rieneke Holman, MS-RN—Weber State University, School of Nursing

Rieneke Holman is an Assistant Professor of Nursing and ADN clinical coordinator in the School of Nursing at Weber State University. Rieneke has been flipping her pharmacology course for a few years, and has developed with her colleague a mixed method research study currently in publication review that compares flipped learning to traditional lecture. Working within a concept-based curriculum, Rieneke's pharmacology course is taught within the first semester of nursing-focused courses. Similar to other nursing programs, her students are coming from classes that have used straight lecture, with memorization and regurgitation of information on tests to evaluate student learning. The first unit or class period is dedicated to introducing students to the course and to the pedagogy of flipped learning. She uses lecture for this first day of introduction along with ample time to prepare students for what to expect with the flipped classroom. Rieneke is careful to introduce the flipped classroom thoroughly, including her expectations of the students and an estimation of how much time students should plan on dedicating to the process outside of the classroom.

After the first class focused on an introduction to the course and flipped learning, Rieneke's pharmacology class is split into 13 additional units. The students are assigned their readings and a narrated presentation prior to coming to the live class. Rieneke discussed several rationales for using the narrated presentation rather than a video-based presentation. The first rationale was to insure that students had access to the content. On this particular campus, students were provided with the programs that the presentations were developed within. For this reason, students had open access to view and listen to the presentations either on their home computer or one that was on the campus. Rieneke also used this format for its ease in revising, editing, and updating. On each presentation slide, she created a "sound bite" that was no longer than 2–3 minutes. If a mistake was made, the narrated presentation made it very easy to delete and record that one slide again, rather than attempting to edit a video. When using the presentation for subsequent semesters, she listened to each sound bite quickly and was able to update individual sound bites very easily. The software's latest version allows students to stop, rewind, and re-listen to all or only a portion of each sound bite. This feature has made it easier for students to individualize their learning pace on each individual slide.

Rieneke also shared her expectation of students to take notes on the narrated presentations that they would listen to prior to class. She shared her perception that having students access the presentations on a computer rather than a mobile device has the potential to create an opportunity for students to take notes and be more attentive to the presentation. She shares with her students her expectation that they be sitting and listening to the narrated presentation while taking notes. It is also implied that the students will be more attentive to the presentation in this type of atmosphere. Her students are also expected to bring questions about the presentations with them to the live class. These questions are to be written down while watching the presentation. These are additional reasons that Rieneke prefers to use the narrated presentation rather than the video lecture.

When first flipping her classroom, Rieneke did so week by week, providing the students with her narrated lectures two to four days prior to the live class time. Through this process, she learned that it is important to provide students with online lectures at least a week prior to the live class. Now when she flips the classroom, she has all of the narrated presentations completed, and therefore can make them available to students at the beginning of the semester. The workload of flipping was higher these first semesters, but became less and less intensive over time. The first time she creates a narrated presentation, Rieneke estimates that it takes her about two to three hours. However, editing the presentation once it is already created takes only about half an hour. Each time she teaches her flipped course, she is careful to click through each presentation and listen to each sound bite for accuracy and necessity of updating. She also mentioned that student feedback about accuracy of the presentations is very helpful. Like the lecture presentations we have created over time, we tend to know which material needs updating, and which material has not changed since the last time we taught the course. This same knowledge can be used to update off-load materials for the flipped classroom in a timely manner. Rieneke provides a perfect example of a faculty member who took the challenge of additional time and effort to create her flipped classroom initially and now enjoys less work in teaching the class now that it has been developed within the new pedagogy.

Rieneke has created a template for her flipped pharmacology class that provides consistency and structure for both herself and her students (see **Table 9-1**). The flipped class template begins with the

Table 9-1 Rieneke Holman's Template for Flipped Classroom

Activity	Example
1. Off-Load Assignments Prior to Class	Narrated presentation (lecture) Assigned readings Various written assignments
2. Student Preparation Assessment	Class Tickets: • Clicker response system quiz • Sharing of assigned off-load materials
3. Question & Answer Time	Students ask questions about readings and narrated presentations assigned as off-load
4. Active Learning Strategies	Gaming Patient guest speaker Medication commercial review and discussion
5. Case Study	Students work individually or in groups—Rieneke is there to help guide and answer questions
6. Review of Case Study	The entire class reviews the case study with discussion
7. NCLEX-Type Clicker Questions	Clicker response system for repetition and solidification of learning with quizzing

off-load materials assigned prior to the live class. Each live class is opened with an assessment of student preparation for class. Rieneke uses "class tickets," also known as the ticket to ride, which vary depending on the content assigned in the unit. For about half of the units, clicker response system quizzes are used. Additional assignment examples include looking up an article about a medication or specific medication or herbal, the most common side effects, and associated nursing care. When these assignments are used for preparation assessment, the class is opened with sharing of this information with the group rather than a quiz. The quizzes and sharing assignments are all factored into the students' grade for the course.

The second part of the flipped pharmacology class template is used for a question-and-answer session about the narrated presentation and readings. After these questions are answered and discussed, the in-class activities begin. Rieneke uses gaming quite often in her flipped classroom activities. One unique and brilliant idea she has for pharmacology students is to have a patient who is on several medications come in to talk to the students about his or her experiences. The example she provided was a patient with congestive heart failure on several medications that students have studied within their off-load materials. In the live class, the patient comes and talks about what it is like to be on the medications and how the side effects of the medications affect his daily life. The patient also discusses the teaching he was given when put on the medications, and his perspective on "good" and "bad" teaching from nurses and other professionals. Providing students with this unique type of patient perspective allows them a real-life practical picture of what patients experience when on medications.

Another excellent idea that Rieneke uses in her class takes advantage of the multiple medication commercials that are on our television screens across the nation. She shows one of these medication commercials and has the students pay attention to several aspects, including side effects listed. The class then has a discussion about each side effect, why it might be occurring, and how it is related to that particular class of medications. I like how Rieneke is using something that students and patients see almost every day on television and social marketing as a teaching tool.

Rieneke mentioned that she likes her live class to be full of activity and allow for students to move around. On example she provided is an activity focused on diabetes and the medications associated. When students enter the room from a break, she hands each one a card that has a symptom of diabetes written on it. She has split the physical classroom into three different sections, one side for Type 1 diabetes, the middle for both types of diabetes, and the other side for Type 2 diabetes. Students are told to read the symptom on their card and move to the area they think that symptom belongs. Then each students shares their symptom with the entire class and why they believe they belong where they stood. This type of activity allows for active learning, categorization of symptoms, application of rote memorization materials, and analysis of overlapping symptomatology of disease processes. This activity is similar to one that my colleague and friend Kat Johnson uses that she calls *"symptom, symptom, who's got a symptom"*. Kat uses this within her pediatric pulmonology class to show students how symptoms can be categorized with the various pulmonary disease processes. We take it a step farther with our advanced practice students, and use these symptoms to build differential diagnoses for diagnosis within the primary care setting.

The fourth part of Rieneke's flipped pharmacology class template revolves around a case study. She parallels this activity to Bergmann and Sams' (2012) in-class homework with the faculty member there as guide on the side. Depending on the content, she has students work either by themselves or together on the case studies. The final part of the flipped pharmacology class template is used to discuss the case studies with the students as a group. Students do get points for these case studies, but as Rieneke explained, the points really end up being class participation points. If students are there and put the work in on the case studies, they get those points automatically.

BOX 9-3 Rieneke's Flip Tips

- Don't try to flip an entire class all at once: flip one or two units at a time.
- Be natural and don't strive for perfection in recording online lectures—it will waste too much time.
- Focus on in-class content, or the active part of the learning. Be sure the activities match the objectives for the unit/course, and that they are application level so students feel coming to class is worthwhile. Get creative with the activities!
- Be sure to have some sort of preparation evaluation. Assign points to the preparation evaluation so students will do the prep work and come to class prepared.
- Utilize content and assignments you already have so that the initial flipped class set-up is more manageable.
- Be ok with a more flexible classroom environment and a learning facilitator-type role.
- Be sure to give students a thorough explanation of what the flipped classroom entails, and what the expectations are, to improve their success with this type of learning.

Each class is ended with a few NCLEX-type questions using the clicker response systems to solidify the content and ensure student understanding.

Rieneke provides a great example for us in her flipped classroom successes (see **Box 9-3** for her flip tips). She has presented her ideas on the flipped classroom at national conferences with a great reception from educators attending. Be sure to watch for Rieneke's publication about flipped learning that measures both quantitative and qualitative data about use of the flipped classroom in nursing education. I would like to publicly thank her for her willingness to share her brilliant ideas with us!

Lory Clukey, PhD—University of Northern Colorado, School of Nursing

Dr. Lory Clukey of the University of Northern Colorado has recently begun flipping two of her nursing courses. The first is an undergraduate course focused on the core knowledge of the baccalaureate nurse, including topics such as patient safety, theory-based nursing care, and politics and power. The second course in which she uses flipped learning is a graduate course on patient safety and quality. For both of these courses, she has created some innovative ideas to use in both the off-load and in-class time periods with her students. She was kind enough to share with me how she accomplished the flipped classroom for a couple of classes from these courses. Being new to the flipped classroom pedagogy, Dr. Clukey is flipping content slowly, still using some lecture-based pedagogy in her courses mixed with flipped learning in only a few classes. She acknowledges that much of her lecture is really not what would historically be thought of as lecture. Using quite a bit of Socratic Method and group/individual questioning during lectures results in a classroom that is full of discussion and more student engagement than one would expect.

Dr. Clukey's first example of the flipped classroom is within her graduate nursing safety and quality course. She has found a well-done video on the Internet that addresses the lower-ordered learning objectives related to patient quality and safety within the healthcare setting. The students' assignment prior to coming to class is to watch this video in its entirety and answer a series of questions using a worksheet. The worksheet questions are focused on the lower-ordered learning objectives and core knowledge about quality and safety in patient care. When the students get to class, they engage in what Dr. Clukey calls a "whole class dialogue" about the questions. Students are then asked to relate the video, the worksheet questions, and the discussion to their own clinical environment. They spend some time in class thinking of concrete examples of how quality and safety is directly applicable to their current and future roles in nursing.

Dr. Clukey's second flipped classroom example comes from a undergraduate core knowledge course in which she teaches a unit on politics and power in nursing. Prior to coming to the live class, students are assigned to find a current bill in legislation that is of interest to them. Depending on the size of the class, students complete this assignment in groups of three. The class opens with a short lecture, described as a mini-lecture in flipped learning literature, with Dr. Clukey presenting some of the concepts and inviting questions from the students. Although she does use presentation slides, the lecture becomes more conversational in nature. Student groups then present information on the bill that they have researched. Once all of the student groups have presented information about the bills, the entire class has a vote to determine 2 bills that they will have a debate over.

The class is split into two groups and uses class time with Dr. Clukey as a guide on the side to develop objective data that is supported by the available evidence. The debate takes place and the students discuss the process of debate, including a discussion of which group brought forth the best arguments and essentially "won" the debate. Dr. Clukey describes within this lesson plan her ability to assist students in both self-reflective and group-reflective processes. She also pulls the lecture materials at the beginning of the class back into the progressing discussion and reflection to help the class analyze the ideas of politics and power as concepts that are intimately connected.

Having a background in clinical psychology equips Dr. Clukey with the gentle ability to make nursing content come alive in an affective manner for individual students. As you may recall from a historical look at Krathwohl, Bloom, and Masia's (1964) learning taxonomy, affective learning emphasizes a feeling, emotion, or a degree of acceptance or rejection. The ability to shepherd students into a domain where they are able to connect with subject matter on a more personal level is a unique educational gift. So why do instructors like Dr. Clukey need the flipped classroom at all? This is a great question. The answer, I believe, lies in the flexibility and additional time for instructors to engage students at an individual and more personal level. The flipped classroom also allows for ongoing and real-time evaluation of student learning that is often not possible within a lecture based classroom, even if discussion is encouraged. See **Box 9-4** for Dr. Clukey's flip tips.

BOX 9-4 Dr. Clukey's Flip Tips

- Don't try to flip a whole course at one time. Consider flipping 1 or 2 units to begin with.
- Flipping a class is a teaching strategy. Do you explain all your teaching strategies to students? Consider explaining expectations to students instead.
- Explain to students how class will be conducted and serve to engage them instead of explaining the flipped classroom to them. This approach may avoid student fear of having to work harder.
- If you don't have extra time to create your own videos, try using what is already out there in video on the Internet.
- Find some way to hold students accountable for being prepared for class.
- Give points for participation to encourage preparation for in-class activities (for example: ticket to ride, mini-presentations or clicker quiz).

Alexandra D. Hanson, MSN, RN—Weber State University, School of Nursing

Alexandra Hanson is an Assistant Professor of Nursing within the School of Nursing at Weber State University. She has been flipping her undergraduate psychiatric course for the past 6 semesters. She originally flipped the entire course at one time and felt the strain of additional preparation and workload associated. Of course, she was successful, and has also been able to revise her course and become more efficient along the way. Her advice to those considering the flipped classroom would be to take it much more slowly and flip one class at a time. Becoming an expert of flipping of the past couple of years, she offers up her flavor of flipping for us to consider and learn from, as well as some of her best "flip tips" (see **Box 9-5**).

BOX 9-5 Alexandra's Flip Tips

- Flipping the entire class can be done but is overwhelming. It would be better to flip a few individual classes within the course at a time if possible.
- When choosing recording software for your video lectures, be certain it has the ability to edit. It will make fixing mistakes and updating videos much easier for future coursework.
- When creating your lecture recording – act exactly as you would act when you lecture. If you walk around and use your hands, do so in your office as you are recording. It will make your videos more interesting, much like if you were actually lecturing in front of the class.
- Don't be afraid to leave a mistake in the video – the students don't mind and have proof that we are human!

(*Continues*)

BOX 9-5 Alexandra's Flip Tips (Continued)

- Don't re-create things for your lecture videos. Use slides for your videos that you've used in the past, just alter for the shorter video version.
- Provide students with a hand out to write notes on while watching the video.
- Use the existing assignments and find a way to turn them into interactive learning exercises. No need to re-invent all new activities. It is likely that you have some great in-class activities already in existing assignments.
- Time is fluid in the in-class flipped classroom, be flexible and ready to fill in some additional time if necessary.
- Remind your students to review the video lectures before the exams as a way to review and study – students in Alexandra's class have mentioned that this is one of the most powerful ways they have been able to use the videos over and over again to enhance their learning and understanding.

One of the main reasons Alexandra wanted to flip her classroom coincided with the newly formed NCLEX questions. The newest question style for NCLEX requires students to be able to apply material to a patient case or problem-based scenario up to 80–90% of the time. For this reason, having students apply material at the higher level of Bloom's taxonomy with the instructor there to guide them seemed like a much more reasonable way to teach nursing to students. Use of class time for interactive or application exercises used to comprise about 30 minutes of class time at the end of a lecture day in Alexandra's old model of teaching. Since she has flipped her classroom, she now devotes the majority of her in-class time to helping students apply nursing concepts at a higher level of taxonomy and deeper-level learning.

At the beginning of each semester, Alexandra is careful to discuss the flipped classroom pedagogy with her students the first day of class. Included that first day is a description of what flipped learning is, how it is different from traditional lecture, and how student learning will be assessed. She is careful to educate students on how to be a good flipped classroom student. Part of this education and orientation includes clearly defined educator expectations of students in the flipped course. Students are taught how to effectively watch each off-load video that they are assigned. Alexandra makes available to students lecture guidelines from which to take notes as they watch her video lectures. In these guidelines (note pages) are blanks that students must fill in to keep them engaged during the video, much like they would have to be during a live lecture in the classroom.

Off-load assignments to be done prior to the live class include reading assignments and a lecture video that Alexandra creates herself. Her videos range from 20–40 minutes in length, but average about 15 minutes. She has used several different types of screen capture software on both her personal computer and her handheld device. Her preferred method of recording has become the use of a low-cost app on her mobile device. Lectures are uploaded to her unlisted YouTube account for students to view at their convenience. Although this is the primary way that students access her recordings, she also has made them available to students using a MP4 file uploaded to the students' learning management website.

Alexandra opens each in-class period with a question and answer (Q & A) time that covers student questions about the off-load content assigned. The time frame depends upon the complexity of the subject matter, but typically takes anywhere from 10–20 minutes of time. After the Q & A session, the students have a learning assessment to evaluate their knowledge base for engagement during the in-class activities. Alexandra gives points for these quizzes. Doing so motivates the students to not only complete the off-load assignments, but also study the material well enough to complete a quiz and be ready to apply that knowledge to the in-class activities planned for the day.

At times, the learning assessment involves a group learning assessment, such as a worksheet of terms. These types of assessments are reserved for more complex content such as schizophrenia. The learning curve of even the off-load material can at times be extremely high in terms of amount of content to be learned. A diagnosis such as schizophrenia is accompanied by numerous terms that are new to nursing students. Just learning the terms can be a daunting task. Therefore, Alexandra uses some of the in-class activity time to help students learn these lower-ordered objectives prior to attempting to engage in a class activity where they will need to apply them to a case scenario. Such a group activity can focus on learning the terms and completing an assessment of learning at the same time meeting two of the educational purposes of the flipped classroom.

Quizzes used for the assessment of off-load learning are completed in a paper and pencil format. At times, the quizzes are graded during the in-class time period if the situation allows when students are working on their own. Other times, Alexandra will grade the quizzes at a later time. She has toyed with the idea of putting the quizzes on the learning management system to be completed by students before they come to the live class. Doing so would help out with the grading burden, but would also require students to take the quizzes prior to the Q & A session that begins each in-class session. The learning that can occur during the Q & A time is valuable. It would be difficult to test true student knowledge base prior to the opportunity to for them to ask questions about the off-load material.

After the Q & A session and learning assessment have been completed, it is time for the in-class activities. Like many nurse educators flipping the classroom, Alexandra uses many case studies for application of rote learning completed during the off-load. She also uses some other tactics as well. The art of patient assessment in psychiatric nursing is a bit different and at times challenging for students to learn. To bridge the reality gap that can occur, Alexandra has found a set of video interviews conducted with actual psychiatric patients. The students watch a video interview as a class and then discuss the different pieces of patient assessment, signs and symptoms, and manifestations of psychiatric disease state that they've witnessed in the video. Next, Alexandra has students connect what they've seen in the video to the North American Nursing Diagnosis Association criteria. The students are also asked to take their assessment and use it in conjunction with the Diagnostic Statistical Manual-IV (DSM-IV) to help them understand how psychiatric disorders are classified and diagnosed by providers. These are excellent in-class activities that help students not only apply their rote knowledge in a meaningful way, but also prepare students for what they may see in the clinical setting.

Other in-class activities include creation of patient teaching materials that are presented to the entire class. In a separate two-class unit on culture and spirituality care, Alexandra is sure to use one in-class session for students to work in groups and create their presentations. While students are working on their presentations, she is able to help each group as questions arise. The ability to correct errors in thinking and help guide the presentations for ultimate teaching/learning capacity is an additional advantage to having students prepare presentations during class time. Alexandra also uses this learning activity for the peer teaching benefits found in the literature. Trout, Borges, and Koles (2014) use of peer instruction in their medical pharmacology course led to higher exam scores and improved student attendance to classes. Szlatchta's (2013) similar study comparing peer instruction to only educator instruction in nurse anesthesia education that grades did not suffer with the use of peer instruction. The method was rated positively by the students, as well.

Other active learning strategies used in Alexandra's flipped class include vivid class discussions spurred by TED talks found on the Internet. TED talks can be found on the TED.com website, where they are self-defined as a non-profit, global community devoted to "ideas worth spreading" headquartered in New York and Vancouver (Ted.com, 2015). TED talks are typically between 10–15 minute video clips by various speakers on topics of interest and debate. Use of this method spurs discussion about controversial topics and brings different points of view to the classroom for dissection and discussion. Alexandra often has students use the think-pair-share approach during these types of larger group discussions.

To help students practice the art of therapeutic communication, Alexandra will use the in-class activity of role play. Students are paired and given a patient care scenario in which they are asked to practice their therapeutic communication skills. The pairs then share their experience with the entire class. A discussion ensues that focuses on what worked well and not so well with their communication approach in the scenario. It is helpful for students to see how

Table 9-2 Alexandra D. Hanson's Template for Flipped Classroom

Off-Load Assignments Prior to Class	
• Recorded lecture using screen capture software and I-pad applications (20–40 minutes) • Assigned readings	
In-Class Time	
Activity	**Example**
1. Question and Answer Period (10–20 minutes)	• Opens with Q & A period averaging 15 minutes, more complex subjects can take up to 20 minutes • Students ask questions about readings and narrated presentations assigned as off-load
2. Learning Assessments of Off-Load Materials (15–30 minutes)	• Assess readiness for class • Points given for course grade • Many times a quiz, but also group worksheets or problem-based learning activity as a group • Use of "just-in-time" teaching surrounding questions from quizzes
4. Active Learning Strategies (2–2.5 hours)	• Case studies • Patient assessment activities focused on psychiatric disorders • Patient teaching activities • TED talks to spur discussions • Role play – therapeutic communication practice
7. NCLEX-Type Clicker Practice Questions (30–45 minutes)	• Summation activity to solidify and assess student understanding • 7–10 clicker questions focused on material learned in off-load and in-class activities • Practice questions – no points allocated • Discussion as a class about questions and why students answered the way they did – learning how to decipher NCLEX type questions as a group

each different pair of students approached each patient communication scenario. The students also come the realization that depending on the patient's individual personality, communication may need to transform. Things that worked well for one pair of students did not work so well for others. The practice of this critical skill for effective psychiatric nursing is helpful because many students are uncomfortable interacting with psychiatric patients. The cognitive standpoint that allows students to recognize the need for adjustment of their communication style to meet the needs of each patient personality is also extremely valuable.

When each interactive learning session is over, Alexandra closes each class with the same "summation activity." Students complete 7 to 10 clicker questions focused on the learning objectives for the unit. These questions are not for points. They are used only to solidify student understanding and allow students to practice NCLEX-type questions. Students have reported to Alexandra that this is one of their favorite parts of the class. Alexandra describes this strategy as a way for students to practice for high-stakes testing in a low-stakes environment. Students learn the art of critical thinking through this process. The ability to discuss their reasoning for choosing a particular response permits learning to occur through just-in-time teaching from Alexandra. This activity takes anywhere from 30 to 45 minutes to complete.

Thank you to Alexandra for sharing her experiences and knowledge about flipping the classroom for the chapter (see **Table 9-2** for her flipped classroom template). Her ideas are both innovative and creative, bringing the world of psychiatric nursing to life for the students in her classroom. As a result, the students have been able to bring learned concepts and skills to fruition within their concept based clinical rotation during the same semester. The theory-practice gap has been bridged with Alexandra's use of the flipped classroom. Thank you for sharing your wonderful insight, creativity, and dedication to the educational process with us, Alexandra!

Melissa Coleman, MSN, APRN—Central Connecticut State University, School of Nursing

Melissa Coleman flipped her undergraduate physical assessment class with a peer after teaching the class with primarily lecture for several years. The impetus to flip developed out of a desire to see her students more actively engaged in their own learning. She is currently in a PhD in nursing program herself. Her research interest is circling the difficult question of how to help students help themselves in terms of preparing for classes and becoming more active learners. How can students self-regulate to prepare effectively for the active learning environment? Particularly with the use of the flipped classroom, this difficult research question is in need of thorough exploration.

Melissa did flip the entire course at once, but she had a peer to help her with that process. She and her colleague each were responsible for their own section of the physical assessment course. Instead of doing all the work on their own, they pooled their resources and split the units up. As with many physical assessment courses, the flipped course was separated by body systems. Working together, Melissa and her colleague split those body system units and developed materials for both the off-load assignments and in-class activities. It is interesting that each had similar in-class activities, but chose different approaches to the assignment of off-load materials. For most of her classes, Melissa would create a short narrated PowerPoint presentation, while her colleague would develop an online module with several thought-provoking questions for students to ponder.

Melissa shared that preparing students for the flipped classroom is a very important step for nurse educators to pay attention to. Students need to have some information about what educators expect from them. Melissa did spend some time with her students to carefully explain what the flipped classroom was, why it would be used, and what her expectations were of them. Another important piece to consider is the nurse educator's comfort level with the material being taught in the flipped classroom. Due to the fluid nature of the classroom and the opportunity for students to ask questions as they engage with active learning, the educator must be on his or her toes. Melissa would recommend flipping the classroom for those courses in which educators feel very confident in their knowledge level and/or own clinical ability.

When asked to describe one successful flipped class, Melissa chose the unit that she has flipped for her physical assessment class on skin assessment. Any educator who has taught skin assessment can relate to the overwhelming amount of terminology and categorization related to the various lesions, patterns, textures, shapes, and configurations associated with skin conditions. For the off-load session, she created a short narrated PowerPoint presentation for students to listen to online prior to class. They also were to complete a few "Quizlets" to help them gain more understanding of the terminology associated with skin assessment. Quizlets are an online mechanism by which educators can enter terms and their definitions. When students access the Quizlet online, they can engage in a number of different quizzes, games, and interactive assessments to help deepen their understanding. Each individual student has the choice to complete the Quizlets in any way they choose.

When students came to class, they took part in an unfolding case study about a patient with a skin lesion, complete with background information, patient history, and the like. Students worked together in groups of 3 or 4. The entire case study was developed on one sheet of paper, which Melissa physically cut into different parts for the students. Once the group mastered the first part of the case study, they were given the next sheet of paper to move on in the patient case scenario. Using a progression of learning objectives, the first part of the case study focused on identification of subjective and objective data. The next part of the case study asked the students to think about important interview questions that should be asked. The third part of the case study was a physical assessment of the lesion. The groups were then asked to write a complete SOAP note about the patient encounter.

The different groups did develop unique ideas and approaches to the case study patient that were shared as a group. Teaching of additional objectives not directly addressed on the case study was possible as students began to ask questions about cancerous and noncancerous skin lesion characteristics. Using the just-in-time teaching technique, Melissa was able to teach the groups and the entire class in a fluid manner that unwrapping the serendipitous teaching and learning interchange that can occur in the active learning classroom. The ability to keep certain learning objectives in mind to bring forward in a case-based learning environment at the most opportune time is a wonderful skill of the nurse educator. Melissa describes this as "off the cuff" teaching, which is another way to describe the technique of just-in-time teaching.

As students discover for themselves the case study progression, they may ask complex questions that the nurse educator did not necessarily plan on answering or prepare for. When these questions arise, feel free to make them a part of the case study up as the story progresses. It is often helpful to change up the case study and throw in another age group or culture, as well. Students begin the case with one perspective, but are then required to transfer their knowledge of the topic to a different age or culture. Perhaps the case study was written about a Caucasian male, but the nurse educator could have students stop to think about how they would apply that same assessment to a child or a woman from a culture who prefers to have her skin covered. The intense and real-time teaching and learning that can occur in such an environment is very exciting for both students and nursing educators.

Melissa and her colleague also used the in-class technique of student developed case studies. When students made the case studies, it required them to have some solid knowledge about the subjective and objective data points of importance. Additionally, they were able to piece together and tease out the important physical assessments necessary in the case based scenario. This technique can be described as the inverse case-study assignment. The product of student-created case studies can be of varying levels of quality. It may be important to remember that the quality of the end product is not as important as the learning that occurs during its development.

The students in Melissa's physical assessment course were surveyed anonymously mid-semester on their satisfaction with the flipped classroom. The student perspective relayed was similar to what can be found in the literature. This particular group of undergraduate students were split in their overall opinion of the flipped classroom at mid-semester. Some of the students felt that it was very helpful and made their learning more meaningful. As expected, the majority of the students were not happy with the new pedagogy. Reasons listed for their discomfort with the flipped classroom rang of their discomfort with a new pedagogy in general. Many wrote that they felt they learned better when lectures were the main teaching strategy. Others were negative about the method due to lack of time to prepare for in-class activities.

Recall the discussion of the average student in our classrooms in nursing education at the beginning of the text. The students have many facets of their lives outside their role of a nursing student. As such, many have had to allow jobs to finance their education take over valuable study time. Others, as many may relate, have families to tend to when not at work or school. Whatever the reasoning is, the average nursing student seems to be busier than ever. Even though the students voiced their discomfort with the flipped classroom pedagogy in general, Melissa did keep her classroom pedagogy within the more active learning realm. With so many potential positives about the method, it was difficult for her to switch back to straight lecture in the classroom. The best quote about using the flipped classroom from Melissa was, "You can see your students learning right in front of you!" The exclamation point cannot adequately be translated into the excitement in her voice as she spoke these words. The best thing about flipping the classroom? Educators really get to teach and reach each student in the classroom on a much deeper level.

Thank you to Melissa for taking the time to share her flipped classroom experience and knowledge for the chapter (see **Box 9-6** for her flip tips). Soon we will be reading of her research on how to help students better prepare for the active learning environment. It will be a valuable addition to the nursing education literature!

BOX 9-6 Melissa's Flip Tips

- Prepare your students well for the flipped classroom – be clear about what you expect from students.
- Flip content that you feel very confident in as an educator. Make sure you are an expert in order to be the best guide on the side.
- Flip for the right reasons – make sure you as the flipping educator have solid buy in and are excited about using the method.
- Keep student off-load assignments to a minimum – be mindful of student time and only assign things that are really necessary for their learning.
- Take the content you taught before and tease out what you really need the students to know in order to meet the learning objectives.
- Lecture still exists in the flipped classroom – this can meet the needs of students who feel that they learn best with lecture.
- Keep the off-load lectures short!
- Use different off-load assignments to give students a variety of ways to learn. Make it fun and exciting for them and that will increase their willingness to complete them.
- Be flexible!

Conclusion

We can learn so much from one another as nurse education colleagues. There are so many ways to flip the nursing classroom. In the previous exemplars, we've seen a glimpse of how different and yet similar approaches to the flipped classroom can be from one faculty member to another. Although I have some experience flipping the classroom, I have learned something new from each of the exemplars that I apply to my own flipped classroom. The value of communication with our flipping colleagues cannot be understated. It is unfortunate that our educator role has a way of keeping us too busy to take the time to sit down and chat about our teaching ideas. Informal, impromptu discussions with other educators are where some of the best ideas for the classroom originate. What if we did it this way – or – Hey, have you thought about having the students get in groups differently? These types of prompting questions from one faculty member to another produce the most rich and relevant ideas for the classroom. As iron sharpens iron, so we sharpen one another into the best educational instruments.

Now that you have an idea of what others have done with their flipped classroom, the ball is in your court. Take what you've learned here and begin to develop some ideas for your own flipped classroom. Moving forward slowly and adding the elements of evaluation to your approach will be helpful to success. Think of an applicable research question about using the flipped classroom pedagogy that needs to be answered. Can you answer that question with your initial use of the flipped classroom? I hope you will be inspired to gather some data that can not only be used to help you revise your flipped classroom tactics, but also help other nurse educators in their endeavors as well.

To flip or not to flip? This is the remaining question that can only be answered by the individual faculty member or graduate student reading these pages. If you decide to flip, I promise it will be an adventure. Not every student will like the method, but every student will learn. As success requires, it will be hard work. However, the outcome of seeing your student blossom before your eyes is worth every minute of preparation. The final words to my fellow nurse educators?

Flip It!

References

Krathwohl, D. R., Bloom, B. S., & Masia, B. B. (1964). *Taxonomy of educational objectives. The classification of educational goals handbook II: Affective domain.* New York, NY: David McKay Company, Inc..

Szlatchta, J. (2013). Peer instruction of first-year nurse anesthetist students: A pilot study of a strategy to use limited faculty resources and promote learning. *Journal of Nursing Education, 52* (6), 355–359.

Sweller, J. (2010). Element interactivity and intrinsic, extraneous and germane cognitive load. *Educational Psychological Review, 22*, 123–138.

Sweller, J., van Merrienboer, J., & Paas, F. (1998). Cognitive architecture and instructional design. *Educational Psychology Review, 10*(3), 251–296.

TED.com. (2015). *About TED.* Retrieved from https://www.ted.com/about/our-organization

Trout, M. J., Borges, N., & Koles, P. (2014). Modified peer instruction improves examination scores in pharmacology. *Medical Education, 48* (11), 1112–1113.

INDEX

Note: Page numbers followed by *b*, *f*, or *t* indicate material in boxes, figures, or tables, respectively.

A

B

C

G

H

I

J

K

P

Q

R

S